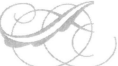

Imagine a top producing real estate salesperson, single mom, bad relationships with men, unhealthy, self-styled dumb blonde… who awakens to her destiny of healing bodies, minds and souls. Meet Nadine Mercey, high vibrational healer. This is her personal story. Reading it will change yours.

Her mission is raising awareness about the potential in all of us to boost our personal vibration so we can be healthy, in loving relationships, and laughing often and out loud. *lol*

In case you don't know the abbreviations used when sending text messages, I'd better explain that *lol* means *laughing out loud*, which we all really need to do *as often as possible*.

— with love, Nadine

Deeper Souls, Less Shoes

An Owner's Manual for the Soul

Overcoming the problems of the everyday soul

WRITTEN BY NADINE MERCEY

COMPILED AND EDITED BY BRUCE T. BATCHELOR

Agio
PUBLISHING HOUSE

151 Howe Street, Victoria BC Canada V8V 4K5

Cover photos of the author by DONNA **SANtOS**
PHOTOGRAPHY

The authors of this book do not dispense medical advice nor
prescribe the use of any technique as a form of treatment for
physical or medical problems without the advice of a physician,
either directly or indirectly. The intent of the author is only to
offer information of a general nature to help you in your quest for
physical fitness and good mental and spiritual health. In the event
you use any of the information in this book for yourself, which is
your right, the author and the publisher assume no responsibility for
your actions.

*For rights information and bulk orders, please
contact:* info@agiopublishing.com *or go to*
www.agiopublishing.com

Deeper Souls, Less Shoes
ISBN 978-1-897435-27-4 (trade paperback)
ISBN 987-1-897435-28-1 (electronic edition)

Printed on acid-free paper that includes no fiber from endangered
forests. Agio Publishing House is a socially responsible company,
measuring success on a triple-bottom-line basis.

10 9 8 7 6 5 4 3 2 1

DEDICATION

Dedicated to all who want the truth…

The angels are talking to me and say to add this:
"Turn the beat around. We all love to hear percussion." *lol*
So the music track to this dedication will be 'Turn the Beat Around'
with Vicki Sue Robinson singing:
Know that rhythm carries all the action.

… also dedicated to all who were part of my puzzle, who helped to
define my self-worth – thank you for being my teachers.
May you find peace and happiness and live happily ever after. xo

… and to Eric and Jaxon, you will always be my angel babies.
Mommy loves you forever. xo

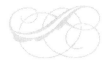

We invite you to visit
www.NadineMercey.com
You can download the music tracks for each chapter at my website,
then get cosy and grab a blanket. Heck, maybe even light a candle.

:-) *Nadine*

MUSIC TRACK
Listen to Amanda Marshall singing 'Everybody's Got a Story'
*Don't assume everything on the surface
is what you see.
Dig deep…*

CHAPTER 1

The path to becoming a soul doctor

Nadine Mercey writes:
In my mind I sometimes see angel footprints to follow along a pathway leading up into the light…. Back in March of 2002, I had a prompt [an angel track] through a friend to keep a written journal to link all the wild events that had been happening for over two years – to connect the dots. Having a record would give insight to my future, although more practically it was to keep me safe and healthy. I recognized the angel prompts telling me I had to take time out of my busy day – my career and single mom-ness – to make the right choices.

It seemed there was no room for error. There was no one I could trust, not lawyers, not family. What was happening was not anything I had ever been taught before by parents or peers. I had to get over my fears. I had to document, to program my body to read the signs in the day, to listen to my inner voice.

It is this inner voice that everyone – I mean everyone – has that they choose sometimes to ignore because they think *there's no more time in my busy day.* If we all stopped to take the time to look at the signs – the answers are *all* there – it will make you stronger, more balanced. Following the angel tracks creates the wealth in your heart.

As long as you are good to yourself and to all those around you, the

1

Universe will provide for you, protect you, and give you the answers you need. You will also find *meaning*: your true purpose in life.

This is my story, about how I came to be a healer of people's energy, what some call being a medical intuitive, vibrational healer, energy worker, or even a soul doctor.

How I got to where I am is an *awareness* that developed over time – over many years.

Listening well to the people in my life helped me realize that *universal energies* do exist. I was shown how to use innate capabilities to rejuvenate the mind, body and soul through light energy.

By sending the right amount and the right form of energy for each specific person that they require for their mind, body and soul at that given moment, it is possible to *reduce pain* and *increase wellness*.

As we build awareness, this increases vibrations so your brain in turn creates cells to *rejuvenate the body* to reduce pain.

What drives me is the need to help others to see clearly and reduce fear and pain, by building their awareness. I am willing to share and teach others to become even a little more aware, and become healers themselves.

By cleaning our egos, we can cleanse the world one by one.

I believe that *everyone is a prophet*. By this I mean that everyone you meet is there to give you clues about your life's plan. It's up to us to figure out what the clues mean – hundreds of clues every day – and to make sense of the people we meet.

Are we here to help them? They to help me? The answer is that *we are all here to help each other*. What counts is how we rise above how we lived before.

Very few of us are taught to believe in our dreams, or in what we *see*.

"That's just a dream. It's just a thought. It's a coincidence. It's all in your mind," we are told by our parents and teachers. We believe those adults until we are challenged to the max where we can't cope anymore. Then we are forced to go *within* to find and trust our own intuition.

It's truly amazing to view what is *intuitively known* by children and many women who have a wider perspective or perception of things in life. We need not be blinded to the energy that is all around us. Energy is always constant, it never stops, it just changes as we interact with each other.

I've learned so much from my children. Eric, my older son, was very confident in what he could see and sense. Eric's ability to see our auric fields dramatically taught me that this can be the basis of our protection. We needed to understand these vibrations he sees as glowing colors surrounding a person, and learn how we could change these vibrations around ourselves – and around others if we have their permission. How we interact with this energy keeps us sane, alive, safe and protected. It's our defense – and our potential. And it is *yours* too. I'm continually amazed how we have linked all the prompts together, and are still learning so much as we move along angel tracks to our life's destiny.

Because I had a legacy of my parents not believing everything that I saw as a child, it took a while before I could understand the reality, despite having clear signs from my own children.

Over time, my two sons taught me so much and allowed me to realize my power. At age seven, Eric showed me how to talk to angels, and how to believe in myself. The more you believe in yourself, the higher the vibrations you receive to the higher power, and the higher you rise above others and the way you were.

It's truly amazing walking up and down the streets when you can essentially read the thoughts of others. I say *you* because I believe *anyone* can learn how.

When we can read thoughts of others who aren't near us, if people can come into our minds and give us thoughts, it's up to us to interpret what those thoughts are. Do they help us? Do they benefit us? Are they warning signs? How do we interact? Do we say nothing?

If you and I have the ability to read the thoughts of others as they come in through past lives (because that is a form of energy) or through people still alive in this world, we will all one day be talking the same language. The language will be no written language as we know it – not English or French or Mandarin. It is universal thought.

I feel that this is important for me to tell others – to help others to realize their patterns and how to recognize and make sense of what appears to be coincidence (which I don't believe exists). The angel tracks are there for a reason.

If we have the ability to *read* others, we have the ability to block others. We can change energy. We can stop it, form it, change it, we can move it. We can get into alpha, beta, theta, delta, unconscious, subconscious states of mind. You can go back to release those unconscious files in our minds that are causing blockages in our physical bodies. We can change the patterns, we can open up DNA, we can do so much with our minds to heal ourselves. We can heal others. We can someday have peace.

We have the ability to get and receive what we want from the Universe if we just ask for it. There is no limit to what we can do if it is *for the highest and best interest*. It has to be for the highest and best interest (and nothing else). Otherwise, if it comes out of *ego,* the energy flow just doesn't work.

It's important we understand *ego.* This is a profound lesson for us to learn. A person's ego is the sense of self (and selfishness) that keeps us from feeling *oneness* with all beings and everything else in the Universe. Although ego may seem to be there to help us, I believe ego shelters and protects our innermost fears. If we have fears, we will not move ahead.

Fearfulness is just an emotion. We either fear or love – it's really that simple. If you love yourself and love yourself whole, you can get through anything. You don't need others to love you, you can love yourself. Of course, it's nice to share that love with others, right?

It is really, *really* important to stay centered and balanced. Your body can feel the vibrations of your unconscious mind. When you clear fear-based thoughts from yourself or others, you can clear (cleanse) your mind of the past, present and future. You can balance yourself and clear the aura and energy around you.

I've learned that you can't control *things*. I've learned to be stronger, centered and more sure of myself. As a busy real estate agent and having that momentum, I came to realize that money is just a flow of energy. What needs to come, you will receive accordingly. (However I should make note that it is okay and I will be able to afford real meat – *lol* – and wear pantyhose in the month of January when the real estate sales are slow in the Canadian cold because it's *supposed* to be slow. And, in case you don't use text messaging, I can explain that *lol* means *laughing out loud*, which we all need to do as often as possible.)

In the summer of 2003, I finally took time out to listen to my body. I felt tired. I believe the angel signs or energy stopped me in my tracks, forcing me to stop and analyze all this. That's when I started hearing the voices and making more detailed notes. I'd been a busy real estate agent for many years – one of the most successful in Canada – so pausing seemed *very* strange.

Somehow I *knew* I would be rewarded if I would listen carefully. At that time, I had many traumatic experiences, strange recurring dreams and sequences of unusual events. I had been unfolding a failed marriage for two-and-a-half years and needed to support myself and two youngsters. Our situation would become tense, with some very unsavory characters, and there would be challenges aplenty. Yet I would take a big leap of faith into a new career and lifestyle path. Looking back now, with new awareness, I realize that most of this was preordained – decided before my birth.

❧

It is incredible how many people have been linked into my journey. All the people who have been attached to this story or sequence of events, everyone has climbed up the ladder. Everyone has gained in their own strength – from *source energy from within*. From their more enlightened positions, these people are paying it forward to those who need help and encouragement along the way.

People are believing in the energy from their experiences. It seems the only way people do believe in their awakening is to *experience* in themselves the *feelings*. And the only way we truly *know* is when we talk about it – understanding our intuition and sharing our gifts, with one another. We do need to get the word out. We do need to talk more and more. The more we talk, the more we are open to honesty. The more honest we are, the more love there is in this world. And less fear....

❧

The love and the peace will conquer the evil. There is true evil. It walks everywhere. We don't understand it. It could be our neighbor next door.

Consider a single thought that is transferred from one person to another, out of ego, fueled by their own fears. That process creates so much turmoil in this world. But we do have the power to come together to battle evil, to battle the injustice that is put upon people for greed – because greed comes out of ego.

❧

As children grow up, family members battle for energy every day, consciously and unconsciously. Your parents, your mother, your father, your siblings. How we battle with that energy and how we receive acceptance from our peers determines who we are in the future, who we become as adults and how we make our day-to-day decisions.

Similar vibrations attract, like fridge magnets moving to stick together. So the 20% of us who grew up in fearful situations, we are attracted into new relationships which actually *increase* our fears.

When those fears become abusive, it's time to leave or change the relationship in major ways. In some aspects, mental abuse can be more cruel than physical violence, since it is out of sight. In my marriage, as my psychic awareness was opening, I came to understand my ex was fearful in himself from desperately low self-love and self-worth. When I finally questioned his control, the communication ended between us. Fortunately, for the most part I didn't focus on the bad. Instead, somewhat strangely perhaps, I saw *good*. I discovered my own self-worth. My love for myself grew. My true personality got bigger and happier as the good came out in me. I was now awake and could breathe, and more good energy flowed.

MUSIC TRACK
Imagine Robbie Robertson's 'Somewhere Down the Crazy River'
I don't know,
the wind just kind of
pushed me this way.
A classic! I had one request on my wedding day: play this song as I
was getting ready. Now I know why – I didn't know then.

CHAPTER 2

Colorful awakening

This was how my awakening first started; there were no ordinary moments....

In the late 1990s, people often remarked that I was *lucky* being in the top 3 percent in Canada for Royal LePage Realty. I worked at real estate with ease, the flow just came without trying. My appearance of happiness and fulfillment at the time masked an intense fear of my husband. I discovered tremendous pain, with severe distension of my belly. Doctors labeled it hypertension, then multiple sclerosis. Every tube possible was jammed down my throat, MRI tests, in and out of hospital emergency rooms. No doctors had the answer. Not even the naturopathic doctors.

I was mom of two young children, with a husband who traveled so he was virtually absent. Number one real estate agent in my city, many people relied on me. I didn't have time to be sick physically *or mentally.*

The earliest recurring dreams I could remember since being a little girl became more frequent and got louder, stronger and reached a climax that spooked me to the point of tears. Finally, in September of

8

1999 at the age of 35, I told someone. The next day at work I discovered one dream – involving a haunted house – playing out in real life. Desperate for answers, I called my friend I had known since I was five years old, pleading for validation that I wasn't going crazy.

She said, "Congratulations, you are finally waking up like the rest of us," and gave me a person's name to call.

But I denied wanting to know the rest and went back to my same routine.

Try as I might to ignore this, the weirdness just grew. I felt tappings on my shoulders, sensed there was someone in my house in the evening, the voices and sound were getting louder. My husband was out of town. Had my father search our house – there were no foot prints outside in the snow.

I spent time alone, found myself crying a lot and didn't know why. Went to see a therapist and finally realized what I always knew on a subconscious level to be true: *I was living in an emotionally abusive relationship.* Leave now, I was told. There's no hope; the only hope is to save your children before your husband turns your children on you.

Wake up! I was being pushed by the Universe pretty hard.

My son Eric, who was 7 at the time, said, "Mommy, you're green today."

I said, "What color normally am I?"

He said, "Red."

I didn't know what this meant. I couldn't google information back then, so I went to a bookstore to flip through some books until I discovered he saw *auras.*

Eric drew pictures of people's faces with the auras, and told me what he understood. Friends were shocked at his level of awareness.

"Eric, how old will I be next month, if you're so smart," a friend of mine said.

"That's easy," he replied. "Just add up the ages of me, my brother and step-sister on May 28 of this year – that's how old you will be."

Wow! From that point on, I knew he would be my teacher. What I didn't realize nine years ago was that this would be the beginning for my new career in the next stage of my life.

᠁

Eric taught me how to play with my energy to make it change. I learned what the feeling was like when you changed and what color it represented to him. Eric taught me to be crisp and clear – it was only a matter of my state of mind.

The doctors didn't have answers. Eric and I did. I was able to clear my immediate physical sickness and thought *if I could do this for me, I could do it for others.*

All of our understanding to this point had just appeared in our heads. I hadn't taken a course or read a book on this knowledge yet.

᠁

Still selling real estate, our secretaries would comment that *your crazy client* or sick client is constantly calling. "You always get the tough ones," they'd say.

I just thought I had the time and patience for them – more affirmation I ignored.

Until people with ailments would comment: "I had a headache and now it's gone."

Those affirmations I didn't ignore. I knew I had something. I started believing….

When you believe you get more. And you only get what you believe.

Waves of new energy, more dreams, this time new voices came. The bathroom shower became my center where information would come while I zoned out under a warm waterfall. My eyes were closed and the water drowned out any external noise.

So much was happening I didn't know if I was coming or going.

Hiding like a hermit, I was comfortable to stay put Friday and Saturday nights on the couch since I figured I couldn't handle any more drama that came my way. I was too sensitive to other people's emotions.

My healthy income slid dramatically to the point of losing my home.

Still, no matter what, I now had a sense that I would be looked after always and wasn't afraid of change for the first time. I knew the Universe would provide for me as it has over and over just when I needed it. Something would come – the best lesson at that time was learning to surrender.

Protected: a new client found me and I began learning about selling commercial real estate. In fact this client was one of Canada's most secure private families, who purchased the largest parcel of land that anyone had sold in the history of Muskoka. With deals of this scale, I only needed two clients! The Universe provided for me abundance of wealth and time to nurture my hidden talents. I could locate and successfully purchase properties that provided large gains for my clients without leaving my home in the comfort of my jammies. For me, intuition and my new Internet connection worked hand in hand.

This position worked for a while until my energy changed again and the computers and cell phones would constantly break down. I surrendered again to the next level of my journey.

It's okay that one person's awareness is different from the next. We shouldn't judge what is right for them. It isn't right for you to interfere – those are *their* lessons. The information I have gathered from other people is mostly *not* to tell them, it is for me to learn by their thoughts and actions. If I need to tell them, I will get that instruction from *inside* and will understand that message before giving them the information. That is something I had to learn with patience over the past months: what to say and what not to say. Most of all, we cannot say anything unless it's for the *highest and best interest*. If I divulge for other motivation,

I will have a setback. I believe my powers or energy will be taken from me. Plus I will not benefit that other person because their lesson will need to be repeated and repeated until that person learns it.

Angels don't wear wrist watches. They don't tell time. They will patiently repeat the lesson over and over, through hundreds of years and dozens of incarnations if necessary. They will give you the signs, they will send you the people, they will bring the information you need to know until you get it right. Learning the repeated lesson will help you get out of fear, one step forward and upward. Fear is what wears us down, that's what makes us sick. The negative energy, that is what gives us the cancer, right down to a cell level in the physical body. The stress creates free radicals which cause inflammation, which leads to disease. That's the energy that stops us from thinking properly. Unblocking the unconscious fears from our minds can make us pure and healthy.

We can choose positive words that can increase the vibration in our bodies, that make us strong through power instead of force. We are then sending signals to the brain. The brain, in turn, can send signals to our cells in our physical bodies to change the genes in our DNA. We all agree that if we learned a behavior pattern we can unlearn it. There is so much the mind can do to heal the physical body.

You might call it intuition or *gut feelings* – whatever term works for you is okay. You can make it stronger. Our eyes catch on some wording seemingly at random. Or, our fingers will point to a button to push for the next song on the radio. The words in the song at that particular time may seem without particular meaning. Yet there are continual signs for all of us. We learn along the way, we learn to analyze little bits and pieces that might not seem significant at that time. What this process truly does is test yourself, test your intuition. Soon you're beginning to understand and appreciate the signs that are given to you. You're learning between a yes and a no. You can teach your body a certain twitch or to create goosebumps to give you the answers to the truth; pain in your jaw if the answer is wrong, a headache or a stomach ache. These are all signs that our intuition will give our body to help us understand as situations are given to us.

I've asked myself to give me signs about what I need to focus on, and asked my mind to store for the future what I need to remember in a mental file – things that I'll be needing to make sense of. So when I ask my mind what is it that I need to know in the future, I am asking myself to give me the signs as I need them.

That might sound complicated, but it isn't. My mind will trigger and go *very clearly* through a list or history of past events that gives me affirmation to an answer that is forming in my mind. I then feel a warmth and good vibration to make the move that is right for me. Over time, I have learned to trust myself. If I am wrong (going against my intuition or signs), the angels will test me, they will challenge me. In the end I will know the answer and move forward in a positive way.

In time, you will *know* when someone is lying. You will know their motive and why it is they are lying. You will know if they are real, if they are true – in your mind. *Inside.*

I've learned to listen to the voices. Some of us can read colors to understand the truth; these people can measure and understand aura colors. Some people can actually see a vision in their mind, like a movie clip or a blurred photograph. Some people can measure the energy, but strangely many don't understand whether the energy needs to be changed or not, or how to do this.

It is interesting how I have met so many energy-aware people. Interesting, I guess, but not surprising, since we are all linked to learn from each other at this level. We can meet on the street and carry on conversations speaking the same language, where others would find us very *different* and wouldn't understand a thing we are saying. When you're ready and the time is right, you'll meet people who walk into your life in the strangest places and those strangers can be the ones who are most perceptive to your needs and life journey.

At a real estate party nine years ago a man starting swinging a pendulum and following me around. I knew it wasn't my skirt or the hair.

He was measuring energy – there was something about me that he could tell was very different. Neil was and is a talented energy worker. At the time he told me he had never met anyone with a velocity level as high as mine.

"What is a *velocity level?*" I thought. "And what kind of crazy person is this?"

I knew I *knew things* but wasn't too clued in back then. Neil affirmed to me just how special this meeting was. We began discussing information, and he studied my intuition. I was intrigued about how he could measure what I was seeing or feeling. Neil taught me to believe in myself to help others. Over the coming months and years, we most often agreed but had our disagreements too. Yet always we worked it through and learned a lot. We understood these chance meetings were opportunities to learn so that we may help people for the bigger picture.

People come into our lives for many reasons. It's up to us to figure that reason out and use the opportunity and lesson. They come into our lives – just when we need them.

MUSIC TRACK
Hear Black Crowes playing 'She Talks to Angels'
Says she talks to angels
Says they call her out by name
This is a song about a person who talks to angels to ease the pain.

CHAPTER 3

Angel talk

*O*f course, some angel signs are not at all cryptic. They can be as in-your-face as this email I got in February of 2003 from a friend who said it just came into her head as she was typing:

Nadine. the bigger picture is coming together. be patient and believe. believe in yourself and what you know. this is all meant to be and will sort itself out. the best and highest interest in all will be met.

A few weeks later on 03/03/03 (March 3, 2003), these next words came into my mind – *angel talk* I call it – and I wrote them down automatically, without paying attention. When the dictation was over, I could read the message and try to understand.

What will happen will happen, you can't control it. You can just make the right choices to make your life a little bit easier – wouldn't it be nice to get through life a little bit easier? We all have blueprints for our lives. We came here for a reason.

What is about to happen sometimes it's not your fault. You are part of the puzzle to help other people learn their lessons. With your patience in helping others learn, you get rewarded by the Universe.

15

You will be rewarded because of your patience – you are blessed, you are guided and protected. Everything will be just fine. Thank you for your patience.

You are loved and through this you are rewarded. Tell your truth. Sit back, things will come to you. You are rewarded now for your patience and honesty.

So many love you for this. You have taught others well and will continue to teach. Love will come to you now and always. Congratulations. Your boys will be fine. They know they are loved. Fun times ahead. God bless...

We need clear thoughts for others. Keen insight and interpretation will be needed. Speak little. Observe a lot. The takers will challenge you. New challenges after the storm. Rise above the mess. You will do that well. You will shine when it's all over.

I didn't totally understand the message, but it felt positive and truthful.

✣

March 13 03, more angel talk sent to me through a friend—

Sit tight. Take care and watch. There are many events taking place that you are not consciously aware of, nor should you be. Your state of mind is fine. Take things one step at a time. Do not put pressure on yourself to get things done. Be patient and listen to your inner voice. It will never lead you astray. Your instincts are all true. Your body is depleting the crap that has been sent to you by the other. And sending it back to where it came from. You are safe from harm. Boys are safe. Yes. Watching – dark people – protection daily.

The storm is upon you. Continue, watch and listen. You are doing well. Keep the frame of mind you are in. It will keep you in good stead. Cheers and clapping. You have learned so much and hence come so far. Keep up the great work. Experience the feelings and remember them so you can help others. You have done well and you will be protected and taken care of. All things are falling into place as they are suppose to be.

✣

The angel talk on July 4/03 seemed as if it was a poem or lyrics for a song, so I wrote it out that way, as the voice spoke or half-chanted it. Some of it seemed profound, some so cryptic and bizarre.

> you're the one who has it all. crystal ball,
> you will never fall from here on end take the time
> to spend time with the boys and your toys to come at a later date
> what you have to know you will
> glow and bask in the light. it is in sight.

> the spirit will flow
> there are plans to show of your future so bright
> you'll be high as a kite
> no time to waste and live to embrace the past so rare a gem you compose.

> the level of trust is a must
> to have a friend to the end
> will create a vow so rich to plow
> the fields of love from up above
> like a dove white and pure
> the music tells all that is for sure
> be aware of the riches for the takers
> witches, will snap, crackle and pop
> when you reach the top
> pure as snow, you are good to go
> tell your truth, you have all the couth
> sweet as a flower, wow, she has the power
> tough as nails. surfs up

> tell your truth, the hard part to follow
> for the parents the events are hard to swallow
> from up above you are watched dear one
> no longer apart, yet closer to the sun
> time will follow relationship to start
> no longer will you be apart
> time is given a space to heal

surreal, so right, so long greed and pain
tomorrow to gain the love you have been given
inside that counts.

tension high for those who fly,
pain and suffering to take place
we are the ones with grace
to take you three to the next phase of life
step right on up to the clouds up above
a place to rest in peace from those who seek greed....

Wow, the angels can rhyme, too, I was thinking. This took quite a while to write out.

delay no more the future to unfold
be wary it is scary the path
that has taken mistake have been give a way of sinnin'
delay no more upon the heaven's door a knock complete

a land that has been forgotten who teach the living to breathe
the strength of God will come back
into play money and greed have no way of survival at this time
what is yours is mine, he will take it away from those who play
with fire and lightning will be our display
tell your truth, it will set you free. believe!

More angel writing in my journal, dated Jan 30 04—
Note the prediction about my international travel to provide energy healing to celebrities.

We have abilities to enter into higher states of consciousness. We need to raise the level of awareness in some matter. We need to make an attempt to understand the overall universal plan.

Spiritual glory is available to the dreamers through understanding and learning.

The day is here for those who fear the light. Speak the truth that is all you need.

Listen to the crazy people – they tell the TRUTH. They are not afraid by the obstructions of the mind. Children fear nothing of us. They hold the truth. They hold secrets if you don't believe.

The balance of intellect and intuition will be your job, Ms Mercey. Travel around the world with work soon to help the famous.

Your thoughts and your dreams, your hopes and wishes are yours for now but will belong to others soon. The path has been cut for you. Congratulations, you have made it this far and have won the battle through patience. The key to success is to listen and watch well. You will be rewarded. Keep it all to yourself.

Your dreams of lightning are a form of spiritual enlightenment – a sudden realization of your personal truth. Something has struck us before. The holy spirit is discharging the tension. Something will happen to change your circumstances.

New automatic writing, dictated on July 3 04—

I wasn't understanding all the advice, but certainly was trying to!

Respect others, continue to work, work to flourish and others to follow.

Believe in yourself, behave yourself, nirvana in order!

The moment you breathe and relax, the moment universal things tend to take place, a natural progression to produce. It's good vs. evil. Evil is as evil does. Not your concern. Transpire to breathe the outline of your contract. Snap out of it!

|Now, this is imperative... lol ... I was getting in trouble.|

Believe, breathe and release.

|This was a commonly repeated phrase when I needed to get back on the path of least resistance... lol|

Strength comes within and from nowhere else. Believe.

Satisfy yourself first. The others will follow.

The best you can do is discover NEW ways to help people with the gifts and talents you have. Channel with purity your thoughts and wishes towards your loved ones.

No need to listen to the Takers. Only jealous souls gone lost. Pasture of green grass in the works for you to run naked. For certain!
[Hhhmmm…]

⁓☙

Angel writing on July 5 04—

Just believe in yourself, Ms Mercey. It's not enough to complete the deal, you must heed patience. No time is required.

Delay the word that has been spoken. Not yet to speak. Freeze, please.

Never cross your legs, Ms Mercey. It stops us from breathing. We like to breathe! [what??? lol – what are they saying?]

We have found in you a place to comfort those who struggle. How sweet it is to guide with trust. Our message will be delivered to those who need it. Because of this you are rewarded and respected for life. Blessed at the helm. What an angel inside. We know you are tired.

Scared are those who fear what they have lost. Surrender those thoughts – that is a must! Be careful of greed, no longer the seed to happiness will it work. The devil will darn a needle with a dragon fly to capture the thoughts and distinguish the lust of betrayal at large. [Wow, some of these angels use pretty flowery images!]

⁓☙

Angel writing on July 6 04—

Timing is everything: remember the ones you love first, second thoughts of those you miss, thirdly remember those who fought in the war for you. Life is a war at times.

Calculated energy in the works for you – believe! You are blessed by many, many angels working against the clock to fix things in your path. Everything in your path that you see and believe, wish to make it happen.

⁓☙

Angel writing on July 23 04, some of it micro-directing my life, other portions downright bizarre, with some strange humor—

Document everything from here on in. Challenges lie ahead. From up above you have been rewarded with stars and stripes, oh gifted one of the Nile.

[Those who see the energy say they see in me Isis love goddess images from Egypt. The golden ball above my head, the pharaoh imagery, the triangle images of the pyramids. What about the shoes? I could go for some golden sandals!]

Government bonds not required. 1. promissory notes, and 2. binding cords. Submission to a greater force, of being bound. Changing conflict into law, and order of the chaos into cosmic order. The silver cord. The Universe expired the entries. [wha? *lol*]

The divine princess of the Nile, the roof, the roof is on fire. Breathe and release. Have faith, discover yourself, the new self, full of confidence and conviction, full of love, faith and hope and desire.

Return to your soul, Ms Mercey, deliverance from evil required. Choose wisely the truth or deliverance. Deliverance is the form of function. Truth equals believe in yourself amongst others. Patterns to be repeated if you are not careful. Choose wisely or deceit will uphold you. Choose wisely: a match made in heaven not yours yet. Transformation upholds you. Believe in yourself and not others' deliverance... [dunno... wha?? *lol*... who's talking here? I get the message... okay... okay... the current boyfriend isn't going to last.]

More dreams and visions. My body was tired. Images of broken glass. Dream interpretations say broken glass foretells loss or damage, changes, break away from the past, shattered idealism of hope and faith, barrier between life and the life hereafter, breaking through barriers, shattering emotions that keep us trapped and moving into clarity to build.

Was I getting the nightmares from my angels now?

Be prepared to document more notes. Transpire your interest at heart. Double standards here don't work with us. You will be taken care of despite your paths crossing. Spend more time with your boys first before play. Challenges lie ahead for the Master of the Universe had decided fate. Here are the stands. Thou shall not steal, thou shall not beg, thou shall not lie, thou shall not keep loved ones at bay. Thou shall not call thy neighbor's wife a tramp. |What? I would never say that. Who were they talking about?| *Crisscross the paths no more. Adventures await you. Sweet, your talents have been brought together in peace and harmony.* |Whew. They were talking about someone else, they just said. Seems the angels were multitasking and have a sense of humor.|

During 2004 I started getting more energy, larger words to string together, and more personal advice.

Benevolent heart, he oscillates his job to work with you. Emanate your dreams. Reverence is necessary, otherwise you will go backwards.

Nirvana is in order.

|*lol*… I'm blonde and didn't get great grades in English. Dunno??? What's *Nirvana*? I had to go to the dictionary… These terms and words made sense just at the right time. They had meaning once I looked them up. Or, I thought, should I ask the angel dictionary! This is what they immediately said in my mind:|

Reverence is necessary for you, MS MERCEY |as they often called me|. *Otherwise you will go backwards, back to the drawing board. Teach them that reverence for the truth is required. Tell your truth.*

|What do you want? I asked.|

Let it go, then believe. You will be guided.

On July 23 04, these words came through—

We can afford to let go of the flow of what is happening, Ms Mercey. Recognition of the potential for emotional confusion out of which can come clarity. 'Your changing consciousness' is happening. Have silence when things are uneasy and expectancy is waiting for something to happen. This is soon to be a time of chaos and difficulty. Help to create new beginnings. Follow this period before fresh growth. Octagon powers have ignited to the highest level for you to exceed the changes amongst you. Deliverance from evil is necessary. Control patterns are over.

[Where did this information come from? Who exactly was talking to me??? Dunno. Octagon powers? I went to the dictionary and wikipedia....]

From then on, I trusted my inner voices to give me clues and messages. I was forced to pay attention to the little details.

At a party, for fun my close friends would say give us a 'big' 'R' word that you don't know. They tested me in front of people I didn't know. Another parlor trick. Without thinking I could give a long word beginning with the letter R that was appropriate and fitting. They were in hysterics with disbelief. Uneducated blonde saying smarty-pants words. Dunno where these words came from – I'd never said them before in my life. *lol*

This was becoming fun....

By 2005 I was receiving medical terminology from my intuitive voices. I had to buy medical books to understand what *platelets* meant. I could visualize the human body cell and hear through angel messages that the diagnosed schizophrenic client was low in histamines in her cells. I began to document the energy.

I wanted more information, but was my physical body ready to receive it? Some nights I would wake up to a strange vibration in my body that shook so much I felt as if I should call a doctor. My inner voice told me to wait it out, that through my power of intent I was ready to learn more. My physical body felt as if I was getting an electrical upgrade right in the middle of my sleep. Do you have to shut down the mind to surrender to receive this energy? Why was it always in the middle of the night?

Soon I began to recognize this concept and welcomed it with open arms. The involuntary pulses were amazing. Could my physical body handle more?

Also in 2005 I began receiving plans and charts as I was truly focused and could keep with the plan that was given to me at that time.

On April 11 05, this message came to mind—

We are about to give you gifts because you can handle anything now. What a gift. What do you want to see? You will see spirit with all the other collective gifts.

On Apr 18 05, my angel writing presented me with these instructions:

Step 1: act out the process in play
Step 2: contemplate life in a different manner, not what you know, but what you believe
Step 3: say things that are on your mind often and as often as you want
Step 4: act on those impulsions you have been given
Step 5: freedom at last.

Ten days later, on April 21 2005 – *lol* – they were asking me to look up the tenth commandment [I'd not read the Bible before]. But before I did, they added this cryptic message:

Weapons of mass destruction ahead of you. Thou shall not steal, may peace be with you. Sad times ahead. Remembrance Day.

I'm confused about the weapons references. I don't follow politics. The messages were getting louder about peace in the world. *And your work is needed.*

Commandment number ten: "You shall not covet your neighbor's house; you shall not covet your neighbor's wife, nor his male servant, nor his female servant, nor his ox, nor his donkey, nor anything that is your neighbor's."

※

At the end of May '05, the angel voices in my head were again very insistent—

No time to spare today, Ms Mercey. Get things done. You are higher. Archangel prophecies are coming straight at you. Gabrielle, higher than Michael. Coming from divine. Now and forever protected.

Congrats, smart girl. You have figured it out. Puzzle pieces in place for so many!!! No concerns. You are blessed.

|Despite all this, I still am human and had some fears....|

To achieve success you must be patient. To avoid failure you need valor. Climb above the rest and don't look back or you will be challenged for a long time. Your challenges are over.

Behave yourself. Smile and be gracious when people, old friends come to call. They will marvel at your talents, be kind. Your talents will be hidden from them now. Believers. Word to get out. Redemption.

|Wonder why archangels don't speak in simple sentences so I can understand them better? Why the riddles?|

In early November of '05, I made these journal notes:

Need to prepare for the next stage in my life.

Need to get away from the past ideas or difficulties.

An angel voice said: *Looking for security before we give you the next piece of the puzzle.*

More dreams: often the swimming pool. I looked up dream meanings on the Internet about being immersed in water: attempting to find inner self which does not need to be affected by external circumstances; attempting to clarify situations and to cleanse ourselves of ideas, attitudes and suggestions by others; transformation and rebirth is apparent.

I would also get interpretations that my spiritual energy was being used up when moving to my next goal. I learned I could rely on it too much as a crutch.

From my dreams I could sense that Divine intervention or interference from another authoritative source was playing havoc at a time when I needed much focus.

Most of the time I would listen to the dreams. Sometimes I chose to ignore them – to my detriment in the end. To learn... to believe and to have faith.

More needle. Less haystack

More diamond. Less rough.

|Now the angels were being clever.|

We have set ourselves external targets. In achieving those targets we may also recognize either short or long term [*both*, they said] that we may need to adjust in some way. I was making terrific inroads to obtaining my targets. Life itself is a school, a testing ground for reality where we are learning to deal with our personalities. Attempting to get rid of old, we are all looking for guidance. We are all teachers.

Sing along to The Eagles at 'Hotel California'
I did receive snatches of these lyrics in an automatic angel writing.
I'd never liked this song and would walk off a dance floor if I heard
it. Now, I get the lyrics. If you ask others, you'll have 1,000 different
interpretations. It's about the spirit world. Once you go there—
you can never leave
There were voices down the corridor.
It's about the materialist world vs the spirit world.
They wake you up in the middle of the night
Just to hear them say...
'*Relax,' said the night man, 'We are programmed to receive.'*

CHAPTER 4

Tracking the angel tracks further

April 11 07, angel writing in my journal—
The beginning of everything. Time ago you were a shepherd in
our fields, designed to plow and reap. Reap the benefits now, Ms Mercey,
you listen to us well. Throwing in the towel won't take place until you
fully release your passions of wealth with real estate. He believes in you
wholeheartedly – receive the knowledge and frame it for all to see. Thou
shall have faith in the unknown, believe. Tried, tested and true, feel the
network, feel the grace of love you have cast on most. Given and designed
to perfection from up above. The holy ghost strives for the most in you. We
will receive your kindness and love and place it for those who need it the
most. The child speaks well of you soon.

'*Livin' it up at the Hotel California, it's a lovely place, you can find it*
here... Mirrors on the doorway, drink champagne on ice, we haven't had
prisoners here since 1959.' Watch, wait and see.

27

[Note: within months I did quit selling real estate. I got to California in January '08.]

Deal or no deal – doesn't matter, you have met your match. Perfection. Idealism, transition, conversation to the max between the two of you. Decisions to be made between lager and ale.

The holy ghost has risen to deal with the path ahead for the two of you. Favors your windfall. Favors your outlook on life in the end. The end is near. Tip toe through the tulips. Trumpets playing to a different frequency. Night owl approacheth. Night owl creeps into your room. Heartache at best. Best left things unsaid...

...'nuff said.

[Note: I ended that relationship – with a man I nicknamed Prince Harming – six months later.]

July '07, angel writing—

Teach me well.

You deserve a break. Hawaii? Is good news. Keeping it real. Keeping it light. California dreaming.

[Note: 6 months later was my first time in California. Seven months later I was in Hawaii.]

10 July 07, angel writings—

The joke will be you and how you deal with society. Keep it light and funny.... Maxed out for a reason to stop you in your tracks to mark spiritual healing, one way ticket to ride. Believe. Homing in on you as we speak. Filling in the blanks. Can't make ends meet is the fear of survival. Switch off the supersonic blades for real estate. No more funding for that is the key. Cut off all ties to the day with the calendar year. Year of the jovial one no more. Priceless you are to us.

[Note: the calls stopped. No one was calling to buy or sell homes through me. I had been top 3% in Canada for sales, then suddenly the deals went dry. Guess it was pretty obvious that I'd better focus on energy work as my next source of income.|

～

13 July 07, angel writings—
The angels speak their mind accordingly if you ask appropriately. Here I'm asking about current man-in-my-life, Prince Harming. He also has psychic abilities and can *talk* to me telepathically.

No reconciliation required for the night has fallen. The love loss is surmountable for him. Based his decisions on others' ego speak, to dethrown the king. Out of context. Out of the Nile. Region is Toronto for the time being. Transition starting accordingly. Moving on to bigger and brighter things. Release me and I shall have wings. Post card in the way. Steeple chase. Hotel California. Wasted day and night.

|Prince Harming is intruding into my thoughts:| **My mind isn't made up about you and I. My mind is all over the place. Need you in my life to sort out my wishes and desires. Wishes leave you and I broke. Desires leave me lonely at the helm. Steering wheel ain't what it used to be. Please forgive me. Nauseous at the thought of losing my baby.**

Angels say, Go! Angels say, never let your guard down with this man. Angels cry for your soul so you don't have to. Angels say, move in nocturnal directions no more. Angels speak their minds where he is concerned. No use crying over spilt milk. Angels need never to leave you lonely. You are the most thoughtful individual that shall be taken care of. Make the grade.

Work to be on the cusp of survival: nurture your soul and you will have it all. All is near. Believe. The outcast will fall. The never-ending saga of truth vs. political battle will travel in other cases. The bonus is in the mail. To each his own. To you, you will have faith that everything works out as it should, forecast is bright. Carpet rides the beach, beach takes it to a new level. |Wow.| *Hold tight, bumpy ride. Bump in the middle of the highway.* |Woops, I forgot my toothbrush.| *No use crying over spilt milk. Wake up and it's gone. Be careful not to put faith in the outcast until he comes clean as you have asked for. Dry your eyes, the worst is over. Pitfall is the calculated one. Gold ahead, nurture your soul and pace yourself accordingly. Sprucely road, phoney baloney no more.*

Love your angelic realm of the king's gate. Have faith in what you know. Proud pappa. Nurture your soul. Folding in the towel as we speak. Keep the wheels in motion.

Next week do as you're asked and nothing more. Placement in your heart still. Nauseous ways hold him down no more. Time to change. Cash out. And run. Run to the hills. Powerful man lowers his crunch. Hit below the belt. Belt is loose. Tied down no more. |Huh?| *Over and out. Write it all down in front of a crowd soon. Healing the pain with ease. Necktie, bowtie, fancy dress required. Natural tendency to fall apart.*

Hi, we are the ones who keep you free from falling. Guest placemat required. New surroundings, old familiar places. Nurturing souls have arrived at last. Reach out and touch someone, nurture his soul in kindness. Nest egg has arrived. Peace, tranquility were what he asked for. Reach out and transformation takes hold to guide him into the light. Have faith. Transformation matches wit with you now. To have and to hold. Transformation hands at the sight of blood. Gore and grief nurture his soul no more. Night shift. Planning attack, rich, wealth, chooses words wisely, speaks calmly at first. Loses interest in the game of hide and seek. Sneak preview. One way ticket to ride. Up, Ms Mercey, believe. The notch has been turned up for the effect of love and laughter. Nurture your soul, speak out, speak wisely, grip the hands of God. Come clean with yourself. Hold fast, the time approaches. Hold fast, hold truth. Tribal council required for him. Voted off? Let's see the outcome of events…

[Note: tribal council? *lol* Seven months later, I did meet Daniel Lou, the first Asian on the hit TV show *Survivor* – he was voted off by the show's tribal council. I was staying and working in Beverly Hills when we met.]

18 July 07, angel writing—

The night has drawn in attention to the mind. Focus is over between the two of you for a reason. Tempted to call to pick a fight, but won't undue his worth. Congrats, you stood up to the man in blue. Lonely is the night when you're all alone in your filth and wealth. Worship the ground you walk on soon. Tempted to call, can't, won't commit to the very end. 9th inning stretch. Yawn, take a bow. Pat yourself on the back. Breaking him down. Won't go down easy but will in time. Ring my bell. Dirty Harry won't speak a word unless you ask him – he tells the truth. |Wha?! Can we bring in Dirty Harry now, please?| *No need to nickel and dime me. Taxed already. Red rider no more in the night. Hold fast delta dawn has risen from the dead and back. Delish treats sweetener not required. Knowledge at best two-fold: one for you, one for me, says Conrad Black. Not entirely yours to forgive and forget. Remember the past. Hasn't acknowledged his worth to you for a reason. Can't keep up with his past. Project the future. No word.* |Okay, one word and I am gone for good.|

|Note: in March 08 I spoke to Dirty Harry himself, Clint Eastwood. Conrad Black, it goes without saying, was otherwise tied up.|

Dec 4 07, angel writing—

TV camera and crew take a shining to the rising star. Notch under your belt. Out in the open where we belong. Movie star material. Moment's notice. Call beckons your wealth of knowledge. Leap of faith, that's all we will say. Moment's notice life to make a milestone. Behavioral patterns repent for the time being. Mocha laka ya ya, gitchy gitchy ya ya eeea. Service debt. We are here by your side. No worries. Onwards and upwards. Leap of faith. Carry me home. Opportunities floating in your door. Onwards and upwards, Ms Mercey.

Wha? Bogeying angels singing gitchy gitchy ya ya! Not quite your stereotypical angel behavior, eh? *lol* |One year later I filmed a pilot for TV, with no prior film experience. Go figure.|

Angels say, *Get a hold of your life and you will have freedom to do whatever you choose. Free to love, free to feel again. On the beach Vancouver night. October man. Nurture him.*

|Six months later I met a man from Vancouver in the month of October. I would nurture him to heal. But would he last any longer than the others?|

MUSIC TRACK
Kim Mitchell sings 'Bad Times'
She's a total disaster in the first degree
A pair of high-heeled blues waiting just for me
This one is left for interpretation.

CHAPTER 5

Ego and spirit, fear and love

April 25 08, journal entries—

Fair warning to readers: I will have to heal you especially after you read my writing. *lol* Much of it is dictated and I often have no idea how to spell the words, or even what some of them mean. My grade 6 teacher pulled me aside and asked if I was hanging out too much with my illiterate Grandma who couldn't read or write English. Yes, she was a shepherd in the fields of Yugoslavia. [Man, she could whistle and command what she wanted.] She was the most influential person in my life: teaching me to knit, teaching me how to reach that vortex through the *I-am* presence. Teaching me then to raise my velocity to give me power to do whatever I wanted with ease. Now I get to raise the velocity of words even more through avenues such as this book!

❦

Journal entry continues—

Most people when they hear that I am a healer automatically think of faith healing, which I have little knowledge about – this has nothing to do with organized religion. When people ask me all the time *what does this have to do with religion,* I think I should address that. Maybe I can

32

just respond that I sat in Pope John Paul's Mercedes at Clint Eastwood's house in Hawaii two weeks ago? Am I more blessed now? *lol*

Clint gave the car to my friend Mike in Vancouver to auction off for charity. Clint is certainly blessed! Hope I get to meet him someday. I did talk to him on the phone briefly when at his house, to thank him, but face-to-face with Dirty Harry would be soooo cool.

Having higher energy levels can be a complication. You have to be patient – especially with anything electrical. The computer does weird things to my files and shuts me down at times. Phones quit abruptly.

It gets so bad that Hamilton Hydro (The City of Hamilton) trucks had to come twice to reboot the power to my home. The stack outside disconnected with the energy in my home – whatever that means. [The repair guys were cute.]

One day the government made a gross error and froze all my banking accounts. That day I was scheduled to leave for 90210 – with no money! [90210 is the Hollywood zip code for any readers who were on another planet and never saw the TV show with that name.] So I've been trying to calm my banker down and let her know everything happens as it should – we can't always see why. It's just worth the wait to find out why and what are these people doing to test your self-worth.

Got to the airport and was fingerprinted and detained by US officials and investigated. They weren't going to let me fly. I had to tell my truth about what I do and it was not believable to them. They didn't even believe my last name was Mercey. Mercy, Mercey me, gentlemen! More investigation. Now they figure my stories are so far-fetched I must be dating or am a movie star on the rise. So they let me in! *lol lol*

To be *blessed* – what does that mean?

To me, being blessed is having the unflinching ability and resolve to share your unique love with others in hopes that they will pay it forward to someone else who cares.

I'm truly blessed to be able to touch the hearts and wishes of many. To help, to teach, to manifest, with or without my 82 pairs of shoes.

It's how you get there – your path – that counts. Connecting the dots, noticing the silence between the spaces. From small town girl, whose guidance councilor said I would never amount to anything, to Brantford's top realtor and snowboarding wife with two kids. Awful divorce. Dating Canada's rock god Kim Mitchell, to horrifying experiences with Prince Harming. Now I am an international healer with a business media twist. [The classic life of a gypsy or witch, some might say.]

It's been my blessing in being in contact with good and evil. Was it to learn by almost destroying my own life? By serving others, giving out energy freely and to receive nothing in return?

&

"Everyone does it in their own spin, in their own time," said Kim Mitchell.

Kimmy and I met at the garbage dump parking lot (the last ceremonial dump as I was leaving the matrimonial cottage) on kind of a speed date on his part (was he just doing his *Rock 'n' Roll Duty* – might as well *Go For a Soda?*). Poor guy, I gave him such a hard time for several years before we dated. How does a girl have a wonderful relationship for years with this Canadian rock icon (who promised her a pair of Manolo Blahniks shoes at Holts), go on to split with him, then find herself touching the hearts of the Beverly Hills billionaire family (who own a top US retail store chain) through energy work in my *bare feet*? How did I get from there to here?

Promises aren't meant to keep, promises are meant to be retrieved. Faithful is as faithful does. It's not the things we say, it's what we do that makes us real. Figuring out how you can keep your head above water and do what you have to do. A leap of faith? Divine intervention? It all boils down to those darn shoes. Fret not – because I am constantly struggling with the whole dilemma as well. It's ego against spirit.

We all need deeper souls, and less shoes.

The ego and the spirit, neither way is wrong or right but you must choose how you want to get through life. How you think – what does this do to our vibration? And our thoughts towards others – how do they feel from our thoughts?

From Bob Gottfried's book, *Shortcut to Spirituality: Mastering the Art of Inner Peace*, published by Deeper Dimension Publishing in 2004, ISBN 0973418907:

- The ego looks for peace ~ the spirit rests in it
- The ego looks for love ~ the spirit gives it freely
- The ego is in constant search for happiness ~ the spirit is absorbed in joy
- The ego looks for control ~ the spirit is totally free
- The ego looks for longevity ~ the spirit is immortal
- The ego accumulates information ~ the spirit is Supreme Wisdom
- The ego is limited by space and time ~ the spirit is boundless
- The ego is only a player in a show ~ the spirit is life itself
- The ego is false ~ the spirit is real
- The ego wants more and more ~ the spirit has it all!

Thank you to all those who didn't know what they were teaching me. Some say: to be a teacher is to know nothing. I say: we are all teaching. You've got to listen to someone to know *what* they are gifted to teach. We're not alone on these paths of uncertainty. You're going to bump into others. We're all part of a grand *vaccination process* to purify the people, the plants and animals.

Your thoughts are your own – so it's your will, your empty space that changes your wishes. You can't believe in something you don't like, so find what you like. You've got to breathe. Then go within and allow the energy to flow through until you involuntary vibrate and allow the power to come within. Ask, receive and *believe*.

It's in your blood. Energy never stops: the old lives gone by, the instinct to know the song, the dance, to sing, to laugh, to cry.

I've found my deepest nurturing instinct in this world is *not* lost. It's just been forgotten as it is in nearly everyone. But we are coming together as Mother Nature is awakening us all. We're forced to ask ourselves: will I live in a hostile environment in myself or a positive one? The choice is ours.

As humans with built-in mechanisms to learn, brought on by fears, we get reminded in our dreams, by people walking into our lives. Opportunities that are presented. We all are reminded with hundreds of clues every day to be awake and aware to bring back our nurturing souls to help and heal others. To help and heal the Earth, plants and animals. Train your body to give you signs and symptoms of the truths to connect the dots.

By connecting the dots and filling in the spaces, we find the inner love, we find the forgiveness past and present in our lives to overcome our fears.

MUSIC TRACK
Tears for Fears playing 'Everbody Wants to Rule the World'
Everybody wants to rule the world
We unconsciously compete for energy all the time.

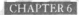

CHAPTER 6

Growing up, competing

To me, it's simple. Everyone (almost everyone) competes unconsciously for energy. On a scale of 1 to 10, with one being fear and 10 being love, any emotion we feel is either a cover-up for love or fear. So if that is true, I learned the following while growing up: it's up to me. Will I live in a hostile environment in myself or a positive one? One or 10? Will you flick the light switch on? Will you stay lit?

"Acceptance is key! There are no victims, persecutors or rescuers," said my friend Tashene Wolfe, in a wonderful book she wrote called *A Path to Wholeness*. She helped me learn there are only Sparks of the God Force who have opportunities to learn and grow. Therefore, there are no accidents or mistakes, you are exactly the way you are supposed to be. You are the 'right' sex, color, size, shape and personality. You were born into the 'right' family, culture and environment. You have all the 'right' talents and abilities to do what you are meant to do. You have learned all the 'right' lessons to bring you to this moment in time. You have attracted the appropriate experiences to learn what you need to know, right now. You always attract the appropriate experiences that you will need to know today, tomorrow and every day in your future."

❦

What was my family like?

My Dad (protective, big *big* hands, eastern block, telling me I read too many *Cosmopolitan* magazines) in my adolescent years would demand [loud intimidating voice], "WHERE WERE YOU LAST NIGHT?!?"

Right away I answered and, surrendering to his unconscious pattern to dominate and pull subservience from me, nervously said "Out, Daddy, I was out and… and… I was here."

So who won? All I knew is I liked to please and help people. I respected his level of awareness.

My brother (this guy was *aloof*, cool cat, non-emotional, everyone loved Mike, he got away with *everything*) would come downstairs that same morning and my Dad would repeat, "WHERE WERE YOU LAST NIGHT?!?"

Mike would say, "Out."

My Dad, "WWWHHHEEERRRRREE WWWWWEEERRREE YYYOUOUU LASSSST NIGHT!!!!!!" [his voice getting louder]

"Out," said Mike again.

Who won? Why were they competing?

My mother – man, she made me feel guilty! Vacuuming all the time. Little cheese with that whine, Mom? Woe is me. She practiced the unconscious competition of guilt. When I thought the coast was clear, I snuck to a corner to do my homework like a good student. Maybe to please her. Then out comes the vacuum an hour later. If I didn't get up and vacuum for her, I would have to pay the consequence in guilt. Okay, okay, I gave in. She won. *Sigh.*

My sister. She was a combo of us all, bless her heart. She is still blaming me for her hardships and claims much suffering because I told her she was adopted. *Wha?* Oh, my bad.

Now I am sure I was no angel in their eyes at times. *lol* I'm sure they respected me for my level of awareness and didn't pass judgement. *lol*

Almost all I knew, all my learned behaviors, my decisions in my life were based on gaining acceptance of my peers, of the people around me.

It was that small 20% of inner growth that awakened me in my dreams on February 14th 1999 – Valentine's Day – that changed it all. The message was a question: *"Where's the love?"*

How appropriate. I was just about to find it. My awakening. My awareness.

The point is we all compete unconsciously for energy. How do words or actions affect our physical bodies? If we are made up of 70% water, and if everything can be measured in velocities (even our thoughts), what does that do to our physical bodies?

What is energy? Can other people's thoughts make us sick? Was I really allergic to chocolate, as the doctors said, when I missed school suffering migraine headaches? Did I really have hypertension, as the doctors described it to be, at the tender age of 25? Multiple Sclerosis? Ulcers?

How do you keep what is yours? How do we get back what we lost in battle?

How much should we give? And when? Do we know that we are giving and taking?

How do you find that perfect balance in this ever-changing world?

Driving up and down the sunny coast of California, I had to thank all those who have caused me to have suffered so much pain and anguish, to make me sick – to be pushed by the Universe to wake up – to see clearly enough to be free driving down the Pacific Highway realizing I've found the truth. I know what my calling is!

There is a talented numerologist who says my life purpose is to *utilize my emotional sensitivity to bring positive, heart-felt self-expression into the world.* My drive to speak may not come easily (and may have self-doubt) but when it does, the words will start rolling. The reading also said that my expressions may be in front of large audiences.

How cool is it to finally reach your destiny, to pass on knowledge, to share from great discoveries of your feelings that may have ran away with your thinking... ah... to dream!

It seems everywhere you turn in the media the world wants to tune into what the paranormal world is tuning into. It's soooo pop culture to be a psychic! On the radio, TV, even the government has psychic spies!

Let's take it a step further. Wouldn't it be cool to understand why we are sick? Are we tired of popping pills and wanting a quicker fix to live longer and happier? Is the world's velocity speeding up faster than the average human body can cope?

Have you ever noticed yourself wanting to keep your distance by choice and not attending an important function, not wanting to get that routine coffee you usually order at your favorite café? Walking out of a restaurant because you didn't like something you couldn't put your finger on? Are we more super-sensitive than ever? Why?

Some people's vibrations are increasing and are sensitive to others' energies. Are they being guided and protected by some hidden force? Are we competing unconsciously for energy? Can others' thoughts or vibrations make us sick?

Some of us may be aware of our natural gifts and are looking for answers and some just always knew why we are here and have been on the same path today. Is it a state of mind? Is one's level of awareness different than the next? We all have one thing in common – we want the truth.

How many of us have been pushed hard by the Universe to get where we are today? You know what I am talking about. For those who keep asking *why is this happening to me* – you will find the answers. It's up to you *how* you receive those answers. When you do receive them, share your experiences to have faith in your awakening, your destiny and fate.

Focus your energy to create a visual connection with your path. Remember that energy travels to where awareness leads you.

You will see some distinct hurdles that I have had to overcome in order to pursue my destiny. The hike wasn't too long once I realized the three paradoxes of life. It's a mystery, don't waste time figuring it out! Keep a sense of humor, especially about yourself. And, nothing stays the same!

After two years of dating a man (I loved him deeply), he told me he had the gift to see as well and read my palm. I would be a powerful healer in one year – a job change. *You will have a student that would be extremely powerful and be famous around the world,* he said.

I'd never told anyone about my dream destiny until that point. He told me that he saw in the future that he would 'allow' me to heal and that he would take care of me because I wouldn't be able to afford this new vocation on my own. This Prince Harming was worth millions in the bank. I didn't get a good inner sense about his plans to control me.

There was a need to guide my parents and family a few steps toward energy awareness. My mother (as timely as it was) complained of eye issues. I booked an appointment with my eye doctor friend. The doctor showed my mother a pamphlet and told her she had a disease and with the prescribed medicine it would go away.

My mother and I had lunch together. I decided this would be the moment I would tell her. My mother didn't know I was secretly sending and pulling energy from her. Within the hour I asked her if her eyes were better. She squinted and tried to bring that ugly feeling back. When she couldn't, she realized 'it' was gone. I asked her if she wanted to get the prescription filled – Mom said no.

I proceeded to tell her what I was doing. She then told me – making it sound like a confession – that my Grandfather would have people come to the home who claimed he healed ulcers and other ailments.

Within the month, there were other issues that crept up in my mother's body. Skin rashes that the doctors didn't have answers to. I began to heal her again. By the time she got to a specialist the rash had cleared (it took about a month to make the symptoms disappear). When she reached the specialist, the rash was gone and his explanation was she was allergic to blue dye.

Two months later, my father called to say that Mom's blood pressure was high and the doctors would be keeping her overnight. I had been ignoring messages in myself that my mother wasn't right and needed my help. Respecting my father's and mother's level of awareness, I let the doctors handle the situation. My father said not to worry and go about your life, she'll be fine.

Days later Dad called to say Mom was still in the hospital and that her blood pressure wouldn't come down. I couldn't take it anymore. I drove to Brantford, and waited for the doctors to leave the room. She had a oxygen mask on and was complaining about a severe headache. Within minutes Mom reported the headache had instantly disappeared. I knew I was healing her, removing the energy that compromised her blood pressure to rise beyond normal values. I asked her if she now believed. She did.

The next morning she was released from the hospital. My mother has since allowed me to send her energy from a distance and allowed me to re-align her energy and help her awakening. My father and my brother followed at their own pace – everyone has a different soul path. At Christmas time, my intuition wouldn't allow me to bring up my news in front of my sister. I respected her level of awareness.

Over that winter, there were other incidents that pushed me to believe, that challenged me not to fear. I had been pushed to the limits, so *surrendering* was my biggest lesson.

Commercial and residential sales activity were drying up. Being a single mom I was concerned but knew somehow the Universe would provide for me. I learned just to *be and live in the moment*, and my financial situation turned around.

A girlfriend tricked me into reading for a group. It wasn't *her* party after all – *I* was the party. Eight people were lined up for readings! I loved it and had affirmation there was a need for me in the world to help provide insight to people. Soon the phone rang more for readings and healings than for real estate. Testimonials and thank-you cards flooded in voluntarily.

For years, the numbers 1111 would follow me everywhere. After watching the Jim Carrie movie *23* (I'd met Jim Carrie back in the '80s at my father's night club as Jim was getting off the ground in Canada doing stand-up comedy), I tried googling to search why I see these numbers. An interesting story popped up with 14 pages of reasons for seeing the numbers 1111. I replied to the web questionnaire and promptly got a message from the BlackBerry of the famous psychic Uri Geller himself. We then talked, exchanging stories for three hours until both our cell phones just stopped working. That's right, they froze. A surge of energy came over me at that moment which forced me to lie down for three hours. When we reconnected, Uri said, "that *never* happens." We kept in touch and exchanged our experiences and shared new energies. He lives in England and had a new TV show coming out.

Uri claims that people who have recurring contact with the 1111 phenomena have some type of a positive mission to accomplish. It is somewhat of a mystery to me what it is that we all have to do or why are we all being gathered and connected together. But it is very real and tangible – I feel this is immensely positive, and almost that there is a thinking entity sending us these physical and visual signs from the Universe. For Uri and I, the number sequence activates the power of prayer, love and determination to somehow help the world. Someday, Uri says, we will find out the precise meaning. But for now he has taken it to show the need to find balance in life and avoid becoming too caught up in the superficiality of our corporate/consumer society.

MUSIC TRACK
Listen to Blues Image's 'Ride, Captain, Ride'
Ride, Captain, ride
Upon your mystery ship
On your way to a world
That others might have missed.
Your journey is meant to have much laughter and fewer storms.

CHAPTER 7

Healing connections

W e are all searching for ultimate truths and our correct paths of destiny. How many times have you heard that if you *go within* you will hear the answers?

Asking that same question to myself, I received a message that said *go to Quizno's for a sub*(!). So I packed up my two teenage boys right then and there, and said we are going out for a meal. They weren't hungry. I dragged them out anyway. Got our food – now do we sit by the window or in the back? Got a distinct message to sit by the window. Don't know why. Just listened to the inner voice – it was strong.

The next sign I received was just that: I was staring at a sign. It was a holistic health center across the parking lot. I told the boys to finish their subs and I walked to that store, took out my real estate business card and proceeded to give it to the receptionist, then told her I was a healer and psychic. I knew I could trust her to give it to the owner.

Three weeks passed and finally I got a return call from the owner. We met for a coffee. Within a few days he sent me cases that were dear to him. We had great success and the phone has been ringing off the hook from word-of-mouth only.

This was the email letter he sent out—

Nadine has the most phenomenal gifts to heal just about anything it appears. Plus she has this incredible ability to gain insight into one's body, mind and spirit which allows her to get right to the cause of problems. If you or someone you know are seeking help with any type of physical or emotional issue and are open-minded, I really recommend her. For those who may be familiar with Adam the 'Dreamhealer', she reminds me to some degree of him.

Oversimplified, her work is very simple; you go to her home, consult some, sit on a couch and relax while she sends a massive amount of love and healing energy into you. One receives healing right away and many times people experience improvement right on the spot.

Three weeks ago I referred an ex-client who is suffering from massive mental health conditions and literally tried to commit suicide the week before. The young woman has made significant progress working with Nadine for just a few short weeks!

Another woman, who was receiving shots for excruciating pain in her legs from advanced multiple sclerosis, walked out of the very first appointment – pain free. She made a gratitude call the next evening saying how astonished she was to be able to play basketball with her son in the driveway.

Another woman in advanced years went to Nadine for a reading to try and resolve some family issues. She had brought 10 pictures and was amazed at how picture after picture an extraordinary amount of deep family facts and details were shared – all without a single error.

I honestly do not believe anything is too big a project for Nadine. Her gifts are truly magical.

This connection led me to Drew who is a very talented psychic/healer. Psychic medium Karyn Reece found me through Drew. More surges of power. No web site, card or advertising – yet booked solidly. I'd looked within for direction and only had to follow the somewhat circuitous angel track.

A fundamental concept is that *everything in the Universe is somehow connected.* This is true even though we can't *see* that connection. Since

I am a very visual and tactile person – remember my craving for flashy shoes – I felt a need to vividly see this concept in my mind.

So I formed my own visual about connection: the party game of TWISTER!™ The colorful bold dots represent people in the universe. To me they also represent the emotional, spiritual and visual. However it's just not as easy as spinning the dial to heal.

If I could create colorful thought patterns to push and pull energy, I knew by building this creative visual I could send positive energy to the awareness and could heal right down to the soul level!

Listening to the thought messages that come from the individual's soul I could send energy to aid or relieve mental patterns of past or present, then help develop their future in a positive manner – if their soul permitted it. We can discard old thought forms of self and make room for new thought patterns to help attain what the person has manifested for their destiny.

I don't use a formula or recipe. The information for each individual gets channeled from their true soul with their higher being's permission (never play with fate) and I connect or release the dots accordingly to what is right for them. The positive energy that is placed makes their being stronger.

A famous visual, from the film *What The BLEEP Do We Know!?* and in bestselling books, that demonstrates the notion of *intention* is the work of Dr. Masaru Emoto, a Japanese scientist/artist who did a series of pictures of frozen water samples. Some of the ice crystals had been created while people expressed positive or negative intentions. Water that received thoughts of love or gratitude morphed into beautiful crystalline structures, while negative thoughts created warped and irregular structures. Even taping onto the glass the words 'thank you' or 'you fool' resulted in radically different water structures. Emoto claims this to demonstrate the positive affect of thought on water. Imagine what the impact of thoughts is on our lives since we humans are perhaps 70% water.

I sat a quartz crystal that was still foggy on the coffee table in front of a client that I send energy to – to help her to visualize and understand this concept. She had traveled to my house once a week for a period of six weeks. The crystal had cleared and I hoped that the energy I'd sent to her 12 brain tumors would clear them with time as well. She can't have radiation or take medication for these sensitive areas. The energy I send works well with her body and gives her a more upbeat and happy approach to life to continue on normally to care for the two-year-old daughter she adores. The positive energy kinetically makes her body strong and she is now able to go to the gym to exercise without fatigue and headaches. Her vibration level has remained higher and she finds life easier with less pain.

⁂

When I was in a movie theatre with a boyfriend, I could hear, "Yvonne wants to talk to you."

I asked my boyfriend if he knew of an Yvonne. He didn't nor did I at the time.

The name Yvonne popped up in my head often, the message was loud but I couldn't connect the dots at the time. I asked my boyfriend if he had been seeing an Yvonne on the side!

Turned out that a lady had heard about me and wondered if I could help her daughter Yvonne. Yvonne had been in the psychiatric ward of a hospital for the past year. She tried to kill herself and was dangerous. Picture a young mid-20s girl curled in a ball, dilated black eyes, couldn't focus to watch TV or read a book, and couldn't make eye contact to have the slightest conversation. Heavily medicated. Shock treatment was about to be administered.

I had never met Yvonne, however our souls met that evening. I was in my living room, she in her room in the hospital. In a matter of hours she was almost free of the dark energy. When I say *almost*, the next night in the middle of a deep sleep, a voice awoke me – a nice voice to fool me saying, "Wake up, Yvonne wants to speak to you." The spirits that were haunting her had traveled to my home.

I had to be strong and brave.... I could hear these evil entities just as Yvonne had when she was committed to the hospital. They got my attention with a rush of tortured sound and vibration I will never forget. There is a reason that I hear and feel – rather than see. If I could see what I heard that night, I wouldn't be as brave as I am today to continue to work with such demonic energies. After that night those dark energies never came back for Yvonne.

Yvonne was released the following week and was reaching out to start a new life! She told her mother she loved her, wanted to go back to school, and began searching for part-time work. The best of all, she wanted me to know she wanted to help heal others. It was so very rewarding to hear and see her mother's joy and for me to know that I was the one who made the most significant impact in her healing. |Note that Yvonne did make a significant improvement but had her challenging moments that led her in and out of hospital. The treatments varied as they were trying many different kind of medications. We are still learning from Yvonne.|

I have three more clients now of the same nature. Alerted by Yvonne's mother and the nurses, the doctors on that ward are now asking questions and are believing the energy that I am sending is not just metaphysical but physical and is producing results.

In each of these cases I helped these individuals move into their center, balancing their energy within a few minutes, from a distance. They were in the hospital; I was home.

It's amazing when a person lives in the vibration of fear, what their true soul says may be different than what is repeated in their minds. Something takes over to make that individual repeat a negative thought. That thought can adversely affect another being whether they are in the same room or not. We are all interconnected |like players on a TWISTER! ™ board|. Whenever you can, catch yourself. "Whoops, that was my *outside* voice." And remember: we must remain light-hearted. *lol*

We only get to change what we are aware of. Get into the habit of practicing to change your behaviors. Your health is counting on you. Aspire (and inspire) to be in the love vibration. *All we need is love, love*

– *love is all we need* can be your mantra and theme song, courtesy of The Beatles. Think we need any more than love? You get to decide.

❧

Like the bestselling book *The Secret* teaches us, our thoughts become our reality. Be careful of what you think. To remain connected to your thoughts, maybe visualize the feeling by saying, "I wonder how I will enjoy that new job?" Or, "I am curious to know what that red sports car will feel like to drive."

❧

Got a call from a friend in Vancouver who got a call from Poland to help heal a woman in Africa who was on her last days, according to doctors. She had tried to take her life by overdosing, taking 60 pills – which had created a liver enzyme count of 800. No medication could be taken to help her situation.

Within two days the count was back to 30 – she was normal. We avoided a liver transplant and possibly death.

I send energy from a distance no matter where in the world. It is usually received instantly with a time lapse sometimes of just minutes.

Sometimes I'm sending energy and don't realize I am doing that until I notice I am breathing differently and release the energy from my physical form. I can ask inside who it was for and usually get the information. I might be talking with someone and not about healing, but subconsciously I have read them and, all of a sudden, will sense the energy changing and release. Consciously I didn't realize this was going to happen. They comment that they feel better.

❧

We are all linked – remember that TWISTER!™ board.

I got an angel prompt to phone a friend and knew he needed me though we hadn't spoken in years. He couldn't speak to me at that moment, and said he was in a driveway on the way to visit a relative. I got another clear message to call my friend again. We spoke briefly again.

It wasn't until many weeks later he realized I had called when he was in the same driveway visiting the same person – his mother. The truth was I got a message to call him one hour after his mother had a heart attack, and I was sending him energy to give to his mother. The next time I called he was in his mother's driveway again, and she was notably fine!

Lots of healing accomplished. Put a heart back into rhythm. Regulated blood, thinned blood. Balanced sugar levels, body chemistry. Got people out of neck braces, aligned spine and tail bones, helped mend broken bones, 3 cases of serious psoriasis. Depression, anxiety and fear. Developed love and devotion.

Brain, pituitary gland, mind focus, increase clarity and purpose. Life force energies, true souls to light. Balance and centre, aligned meridians. Emotional release, past life, this life, in all the different mind sets and brain awareness. Increased mind awareness, built safe places for souls, transition to help manifest next stage in their life force. Build confidence.

Family counseling: a whole family, grandmother and her two generations to help evolve and understand.

Mending fences of mother and daughter issues. Mother thought her daughters had a problem. Brought the talents out of the daughters and helped the mother with issues she never knew she had around kindness and clarity. Helped others to speak to lost loves ones. Brought in new spirit guides, got rid of old ones. Removed thought forms, old habitual patterns.

Channelings through writings are unique and detailed. The unique wording that the individual would use or perhaps a meaningful phrase of a lost loved one would occur, giving affirmation for them to believe.

MUSIC TRACK
Jackson Browne singing 'Doctor, My Eyes'
I have done all that I could
To see the evil and the good without hiding
... Was I unwise to leave them open for so long
... Is this the prize for having learned how not to cry?

CHAPTER 8

Learning and teaching healing

id you know what the word *doctor* means, its root meaning? It comes from the Latin verb *docre*, meaning to teach. Apparently the earliest use of the word in written English was in 1303, but the term applied to doctors of the Church, meaning learned ones in the spiritual realm. It was not until 1377 that it was used in the sense of a physical doctor who treats illnesses or diseases.

I'm not a medical doctor although in my readings I do get specific medical terminology. Since I don't have a science background, I had to buy a nursing dictionary to discover what information was coming through me. In my healings I found it wasn't necessary to be articulate and educated in medical science, I just need to send energy to the patterns I formed in my mind. Sometimes the information was rather serious, yet I automatically knew how much and what form of energy and how frequently I should send the energy. I could read how well the client was receiving it and any movement in the energy. Did it leave the physical body? Did the energy transfer to another location in the body? Any pressures I needed to release?

Sometimes, on the contrary, the information given to me is very clever and witty, and not about diseases. For example, my girlfriends are

51

amused by my abilities. They said to 'read your boyfriend problems.'
I went within and got the terminology: *urologist*. I pause and waited
quietly in myself for the next part of the message (thinking it's a serious
medical problem). Next came the message: *a urologist is not required for
that man. He's pissing in the wind!* followed by the sound of laughter.

Seriously: after the hundreds of testimonials, I still wake up every
morning and ask is this really happening to me? But I don't question
what I need to know as far as my level of education or whom I have
studied under. The healings are all unique to themselves. It's their soul
and angel guides that tells me what to do. The intent to help is strong,
the belief is real, and the satisfaction is in my heart.

I just wish I could share this energy with many, many more – and
that they will then share the energy and pay it forward to others who
want it.

Some of my clients are experienced healers who see energies themselves. They have told me several things, including that I work with
the three archangels, who are with me. I've heard that I am in such
and such dimension, that orbs and fairies are in my house, that my
energy is divine but also from other planets. It's all new for me and I
am sure I have a lot to learn and to teach. What matters to me today is
that in each situation I be in the state of mind to shut everything else
down than interferes, so I can be accurate enough to raise my vibration
as high as I can to help others. Everything else doesn't matter, who or
what I am.

What's a healing like? Could you do it yourself? First I ground and
center the individual and his or her energy. Next I prepare, putting
in positive energy to prepare the client, before beginning to push and
pull the adverse energy. It's like I am the big black fellow in the film
The Green Mile who takes away the bad energy. I release what a person
can't and pump them up with so much positive from the Earth and
the Divine that they begin to release themselves. Usually a client will
feel good instantly, though sometimes sleepy yet with lots of energy. A
person may have one day of shut down and the next they are feeling

renewed. Sometimes energy works with them for only a few days, depending on their illness.

The mind is an ultimate endless source of wellness. Are you ready to explore yours?

Back when my son Eric was 7 years old, I had told him to stay out of the cookie jar so he wouldn't spoil his appetite for dinner. As I was upstairs, I heard a scream from Eric downstairs. I ran down to find out that he was terrified and angry with me.

"Why?" I asked.

"For sending Bellum down to get me out of the cookie jar," he said defiantly.

I said, "Who and where is Bellum?"

He pointed and said, "It wasn't funny to do that, Mommy! She scared me."

I asked who that was, and he said *your angel*.

Eric drew an outline of descending angels and matter-of-factly stated who they were and what their jobs were. Bellum is pink and light blue. I asked how he knew this and he told me he *spoke* to the angels.

I asked Eric if Mommy could too and he said simply *yes*.

"How, Eric?"

"Just *ask*," was his answer.

Anxious as I was, it took a long time to accomplish some sort of connection with an angel. First he told me they were often pink and sparkly. Eric and I sat on the couch in silence, with me half-closing and squinting my eyes desperately, waiting for answers. At length he said, "Only when you're ready, Mommy. They want you to be patient. Angels don't wear wrist watches."

Eric could get answers to almost anything (anything that they felt safe to tell him at his tender age). He could visualize himself in the middle of a circle of angels and call out to the one who would help him for the specific task at hand. When he became older and played soccer, Eric would call in a spirit to help him tend goal. He knew that normally he might not jump high enough to reach a difficult speeding ball. He knew what to do to bring in what he called *the power* to guide him in doing his very best in that situation.

Gradually Eric taught me to *hear* the messages and to write them down. At first it was nursery rhymes, then nicknames of people were given. I asked Eric why, and he said for your protection. Not to give people air space so they could tap into your energy. Smart. Or clever. This kid was amazing.

I received an analogy: the story of *Goldilocks and the Three Bears*. Over and over repeated like a recurring dream. (Causing me to wonder if there is any difference between dreaming during the day or night.) I had golden hair that was curly. Wait a minute: I had three men in my life that I was trying to decide which one to settle with! *lol* Then the analogy went away. So did the bears. "This one is too hot." "This one is too cold." "This one is just right." Except – let's just say he wasn't my Mister Right. He was my Mister For Now. Since then the rhyme and rhythm in my personal life has changed.

The rhymes progressed to stories, to larger pages and pages of predictions and writings. Some people call this *automatic writing*. The content was for me, or for anyone. When I started into the healing work, I began receiving medical terms and images of a body's internal workings.

What was very curious were third-party writings that were received without asking – these are messages for me sent through another psychic! Donna was and is a client who came for one energy session to experience my work. It is so bizarre what happened next, that I am still amazed. Donna began to get automatic messages to pass on to me, which she did via email. They appear just in time to guide me. The best line to describe what we all go through including myself is *we can't always see past the choices we haven't yet made*. Donna receives messages with *great* detail at the precise moment before the event happens, to direct me quickly. When the advice is in writing I seem to listen to the message far better than if Donna simply told me. So why Donna and not another psychic girlfriend? Simply because she was chosen at this time. Who is she talking to? Donna's messages are signed at the bottom *Gabrielle*. Was this to be my main angel/guide?

Here are two of Donna's emails, the first after her initial healing session with me, and the second which had the first dictated message from Gabrielle—

Hi Nadine, I was in the process of writing to you when I opened my email in-box and saw your note! lol

I just wanted to let you know how absolutely blessed I feel to have you right at my fingertips! The energy I felt moving through my veins today was absolutely incredible. I feel very peaceful and very good, however, I feel something very peculiar – somewhat of a void, which I know is somehow connected to the peace I feel. Whatever it was, it couldn't have been that important to my well-being, because I'm doing just fine without it! lol

I somehow feel that you were brought into my life to get my soul in shape to allow me to do what I must do. And I feel 'advised' that you are the only person that can work with me. You're probably more capable of communicating with my spirit guides than I am, so chances are, they told you more than they tell me! I'm sure they think I'm illiterate!!!! hehehehe

I try not to get too deep with people in spiritual conversation, since I feel that my main purpose is just to make them laugh... and when I start talking about connecting to a higher energy source, etc., they just look at me strange... and don't laugh anymore... lol However, I really don't know what I would be without my angels and guides comforting me and directing me.

I have great faith in your abilities to align me both spiritually and physically, which will result in my ability to see my path a lot clearer. My mind is very clear tonight, my energy level is higher than it's been for years. I'm going to study for my flight test until midnight – the first time in 2 months! Like I said earlier, I feel like there's something missing, just don't know what it is – just know I really don't need it back! lol

Nadine, I believe you're a rare gift... you're akin to Rapid Lube & Suds for the soul, a person where guides and angels can bring their sorry little souls for healing, revitalization and redirection! You are truly wonderful!

I sure look forward to seeing you again and I anticipate feeling even better over the next few days!

Thanks again, Nadine,

ttys

Donna

After sending me that first email, and Donna asking for more wisdom, she got just that! Donna began writing what she *saw* and also what was *dictated* to her to help guide me—

I can feel some very great things for you, Nadine... some absolutely amazing things... I actually just visualized you getting into a black car... a nice black car, holding hands with a real hunkaroo... real hunky... and a huge diamond on your hand... wow... that was weird. But very nice car, something nicer than a Mercedes or Beamer, it's like a Jag or Porsche. Perhaps an athlete... looks like one of those guys in the underwear commercials... nice car with a console... you were smiling from ear to ear... (geesh... that was a crazy little trip... *lol* I am now putting my crack pipe down... *lol*)

[And the angels dictated to her—] *To our precious guide Nadine: You are to remember that all things in your life have various streams to fruition. It's always a test. If you allow certain vibrations to intercept yours, your great and important abilities, which have been given to you, will be compromised or worse yet, robbed and diminished.*

We have great faith in you, and you will be justly rewarded. Your gifts are to be given generously to those who need and charged to those who think they need them, yet have no idea how much they don't need them.

All things behind you, are behind you and serve no purpose to you today, aside for the fact that you have gained great wisdom and confidence in the powers above. There is absolutely no power in your close vicinity that can harm you, even though it may seem to you that this is possible. Smile and wish well. You are protected.

When the word power *is said, it is to mean the willingness and the humble way in which you allow communication through yourself for the betterment of all those we send to you. You are a wise little hen. You are not to worry about affairs of the heart. We will look after you in ways that you cannot even imagine, if you stay true to us. You will not be without love, we will give you everything you need. You must grow and become more confident and we will be there for you.*

You must be smart in business and earn all that is necessary for you to continue our work. We will make sure that the opportunities are there. You must beware of wolves in sheep's clothing, for we don't take lightly to our works, via you, being capitalized on. Many people will want everything that you can give them, but you know there are things that we don't want you to give people, for it will truly interfere with their own personal lessons. A person cannot live saying Life sucks, Life sucks, Life sucks, Woe was me, Woe was me *and get healed. That person needs to truly want change.*

Donna has questioned us about 'Prince Harming' and we are saying to you directly, that this person has no power over you. He has never had power aside from the heart and the hopes and dreams of an easier and better life. But, we say to you that you are not made of this fiber, or we would never have chosen to bring you into the circle. You fear not the decisions of the past, for they are dust upon the ground. Today is the day you must worry about. Hurdle the little obstacles, and give true love and compassion to your foes. You may represent power to many, but they know little about true power.

We have offered you a job and you have accepted. You must bring it to as many people as necessary, and spread the word of enlightenment. The people who are enlightened, will go away more enlightened, however, the people who may be skeptic, will go away believing that we are here. They will for the first time believe in a much higher power and it will change their life forever. We are here today to change the hearts of the world for the betterment of mankind. It is our desire. You know how to get a hold of us.

Gabrielle, Jonathan et al.

Interestingly enough, Prince Harming pops up into my dreams that night, sending me roses and seeming pleasant in the dream. Knowing what I know on this plane to be the opposite and I would be foolish to go backwards [Hey, jets don't have rear view mirrors], my question was: *If we are all born divine, then is there such thing as dark energy? What is dark energy?*

Without me consciously calling Donna, that morning she replied with an answer—

You are good, Nadine, and they are happy that you have truly awakened and realized your talents and role in this plane. You will do exactly what you're suppose to do, more and more each day, because you will start to function on a different brain pattern and your animalistic tendencies will become less and less. Healing is your path and as you heal, more people will be enlightened. One will be by their experience and the other will be by their testimony and true belief that they are both responsible for their ailments and they are capable of correcting their ailments. Yes, there may be medicines that can help them but this simple exercise of having people understand just how powerful they are as individuals is very important to global growth.

Donna is of the belief that the Dark is the Dark, but we are saying at this time that the Dark is simply dark/light and the Light is simply light/dark. Our goal is to have perfect balance. We cannot expect everyone on Earth to be dancing around and we certainly cannot say that darks cannot do all the things that lights can do. You share the same space. All have souls. You are doing the things you should be doing. You will know above all what is right and what is wrong for you.

Your healing will be viewed by skeptics as something that is not good, but what isn't good about feeling better? It is important that persons with ailments realize that we did not do those things to them, they allowed themselves to become that way by the inability to detach from the things that they thought were of value. You will be able to tell people how to make sure they keep tuned up, because we don't expect you to have to continue to fix the same car over and over and over.

They must learn themselves how to manage the ship. You will be able to tell them exactly why they are in this condition, whether it be a relationship or a situation at work that they are not addressing. You will be able to help them make life choices that will prevent them from sitting on your couch week after week after week. You know the lessons of weekly releasing and tuning up on a basic level, which will allow people to manage their lives to prevent ailments. We would like you to write a book called An Owner's

Manual for the Soul. *Do not worry about the tribulations in your life because they will serve as testament.* Donna *keeps wanting to write classes, but we are saying seminars called* Soul Search; *she is a very difficult person to get through the brain waves of. Her mind is all over the place. But she is open and available. She is a delinquent child.*

All will be well, Nadine, and we are with you on your journey. You are doing much good and will be enlightening more and more each day. The book and seminars are important because they will reach more people and a good portion of the proceeds will be distributed to... her mind is at work again... lol... a charity which will allow people, mainly women, to look good and feel better and have much more control over their life.

That's it for now because Donna is being difficult.

Always with you, Gabrielle et al

Have you been searching for an open-minded medical doctor? One who has some knowledge of how your beliefs affect your health? If you have one, please let me know through my website at www.NadineMercey. com, so we can share the names of some of these modern pioneers of integrated medicine.

MUSIC TRACK
Jesus Jones performing 'Right Here, Right Now'
Right here, right now
There is no other place I want to be
Right here, right now
Watching the world wake up from history

CHAPTER 9

Indecision

One fear I had was making my financial commitments with this transitional position I was entering (i.e. phasing out of real estate sales and devoting myself full-time to energy healing).

What I discovered was that my ego was not well refined. When attacked and persuaded by the egos of my Ex and my latest boyfriend Mike, I was a mess, and it was like I was standing at a toilet, flushing money down it. A day turned into a week, turned into a month, and I wasn't making money. I was scrambled because Mike was telling me I didn't need all of my stuff, while Prince Harming was telling me I didn't deserve all of his stuff and I was going to be penniless. And my ego was dialing 911.

My own negligence, by allowing the thought processes of these other egos to interfere with my own ego, resulted in me essentially selling the farm, downsizing, wasting three whole years financially. I was doing paperwork that should have only taken me a month to do and selling a handful of houses, because I was on a super pity party. If I could rewind the movie, I would want myself focused, taking the bull by the horns, selling 50 houses a year and getting on with life. Though I failed in some ways, I was learning a lesson about indecision.

How did this happen? So many people were saying, *How are you going to do this?* My debt owed to Revenue Canada looked huge to Mike. However, that was peanuts to a seasoned, good realtor. I could have just worked and paid it off, instead of chewing up a couple of years fighting it. At the end of the day, I settled with the revenue folks, borrowing heavily against my mortgage for the tax debt and for start-up money for a new career. Matter of fact, I wasted so much time and angst about taxes and financial worry – how ridiculous is that!

The lesson I learned was this. Some people may perceive the foothills in my life to be as big as the mountains in theirs. Mike couldn't understand this and here I was listening to someone who couldn't understand my skill set and motivation.

Now, the underlying element here is my inner voice, pushing me or calling me to help mankind. A voice that says, *We have given you many riches. Please return the favor to mankind. Go where most will not go. Help where many will not help. Rise above the norm and make a difference.*

So, my head spins. I have two, sometimes three kids (my sons and a step-daughter) to be a mom to. So, I know the time to fly the coop is not now. Now is a time to prepare for the move completely and effortlessly to the next level.

I am always given things in the form of metaphors, to ease my mind about the path I must take. If I was in university, taking my Bachelor of Science degree, I would need a particular set of subjects to graduate. I would not be able to take my Masters degree until I had all of the prerequisites. Then, before I was to take my Masters, I would have to write a test which would cover all of my general and specific knowledge. I would not be able to move forward unless I fulfilled these requirements.

Similarly, in life, there are no shortcuts. There's no hidden shorter path. The subjects must be learned in life as in the other systems we have in place to travel through life. There's no one in that university classroom who can say, *Hey, hey, I'll do your classes for you.* Or a place you can buy your school credits. There's no easy way. The systems we have in place in the material world, are simply copies of systems in place elsewhere. You either learn the stuff, and pass... or repeat, repeat and repeat.

❧

This email from Donna was off the charts for me! The detail was uncanny to me... ooohh, sppoookkky!—

Good Morning, Nadine!

I miss having time to talk to you! Always so much to think about and do. I don't know about you, but my life is always so different every single day. I am a stranger to normality, and schedules... lol

Sometimes I think I'm letting my life down, simply because I can't prioritize correctly. But then if you look at it like it's all a game, it would appear that I have to work on my strategy. I think our lives are parallel in a lot of areas and perhaps by organizing these messages for you, I will gain insight into my own game plan... lol

The information I get for you has been very scrambled as of late. Very scrambled and I think that aspect is information in itself. I couldn't figure it out. Here are three analogies which you will be able to understand and I'm letting this flow now....

1) You have a ball of yarn, a pair of knitting needles and a pattern – and someone wants you to knit them a sweater. You know exactly what to do, but everyday, they make a change in the pattern, they want a different color. And worse yet, they keep messing up the ball of yarn. You know what you have to do. However, they are insecure in their thoughts, which makes your job impossible.

2) You and a friend are taking a small road trip. You're traveling from Ancaster to Dundas. You tell your friend to go to Wilson Street, to travel down Wilson Street and turn left on Main Street – which will take them right into Dundas. They talk to a friend, who tells them that the fast route is Highway 403. They will then simply take the Aberdeen exit, turn left on Longwood and turn left on Main Street, then if they want they can take Cootes Drive or stay on Main Street. The choice is theirs. They decide to ignore your advice and take the advice of the friend – because it's faster – and the end result should be the same. Not only that, they actually believe that since the friend has been around a bit longer, they know better. In

15 minutes, you're in Dundas, waiting for your friend. Who is lost, and calls you from somewhere around St. Joe's Hospital. Your friend is not where you expected them to be, because they did not stay on the prescribed path. And now, you have to give them twice the amount of directions to get them to their destination. Or perhaps even go find them because they are lost, and had they followed your directions, this would never have happened.

3) You are a doctor and your patient has been very sick. You keep running tests, and diagnosing her ailments, and making her a priority because she's a woman of substance in the community. Sometimes other patients have to wait hours, while you try to assist this Queen-like woman. The other patients understand and sit patiently. You certainly don't want to upset this woman. You view her as a higher life form than you, when in fact you, her and all the other patients are exactly the same life form. Then, one day, you discover that this Queen-like woman is not only self-destructing, living a self-destructing life, but is also visiting a lot of other doctors and wasting a lot of your time which would have been better spent on those who really needed your services and were patient enough to wait.

Prioritizing is the lesson here today. Filtering and priorities. Remember, the blood of Earth flows with money, that is the currency of life. Without money or gold wafers, voices are not heard, success is not deemed, works are not done. Money is man-made, thus all of mankind can manifest this. Money requires a route to get to you, meaning that you just can't conjure it up; it needs a path to travel. There is a money flow, which can certainly be manifested, certainly conjured up. Take every opportunity to make good business. There is plenty of time to make money and do good things.

Do not waste your time on perceived wealth. Even snakes can slither into a gold bracelet and look expensive, but at the end of the day, it's still a snake. Some people have a surplus of gold wafers and would love to buy enlightenment – but there are no enlightenment stores. Some people have a surplus of enlightenment and would love to buy an abundance of gold wafers, but you can't buy gold wafers with simple enlightenment – there must be supreme balance. Do not get blinded by a patient coming in with a stack of gold wafers. They cannot buy enlightenment, nor will they find their way to Dundas if they do not follow the prescribed route.

There are things that must be dealt with today, even if today happens tomorrow.

Directions. As you read this, look around for a piece of paper and pen. Now, that you have it, think about people and their problems. Think about the biggest concerns that people have when they come to see you and the biggest messes they have made with their life. Only the biggest problems. Now, write down these 12 problems. Now, jot down in one line, the answer to these problems. These will be chapters of your first book. Do not stray from these problems. They are the Problems of the Everyday Soul, and the Soul's Guide to overcome these obstacles. Do not worry about writing a good book, there are many that have talents. You must put this stuff on paper, the rest will look after itself. You didn't do all that well in English; we know others that did! lol

There will be other Guides, but this is primary.

Okay, Nadine, descramble and prioritize. Earn money, have fun, and grow.

With love and care, Gabrielle et al

I made a list to set priorities. I really needed to get this sorted out.

1) I must provide myself and my family with food and shelter. *To do so I must work.*

2) When I work, I must pay expenses to work and pay taxes and own a car. *To do so I must make payments.*

3) I must provide myself with outside interests. *To do so I must work to afford it. Thus, I must pay more expenses, and work and pay more taxes.*

4) I must provide my soul with space. *I cannot work during this time, so I must work more effectively other times.*

5) I must reach my goal that I want to help save the world in the future. *Which means I must use every minute of every day to either work or provide my soul with space. Today.*

If I take work out of this equation, I have a mess. *lol* A starving mess! *lol*

Care must be given that we don't try to manifest things we can't manifest easily. Manifest happiness, good people, beauty, ease of living, and block out all people who wouldn't donate a kidney to you today. *lol*
    We must stopping asking *Why*… and just do. Work like you've never worked before, helping people in life like never before. A person in university doesn't ask the silly questions that kids in grade school ask. Gaa Gaa Goo Goo – is simply baby talk. Regardless what is happening tomorrow, or next month, or in the next decade, the truth of the matter is we are in the university of life and must do our work and not worry about what they're learning elsewhere. We can get a tutor but we can't spend our time worrying about other things. We must work on our own subjects. We know what they are!

From Donna—
    I think this letter will have some importance to you. *Look straight ahead. You are the driver of your own ship. The waters may be smooth, or they may be choppy. It may even be a storm. Just keep on going straight ahead. North America wouldn't have been discovered if people did not battle the storm.*
    People are winning over the storm every single day, we can too!
    ttys, Donna

I had been guiding a client and felt it necessary to take a step back as they were being challenged by outside influences and needed to see clearly on their own. There was nothing I could do at that time. Along comes Donna to mend my heart as below [remember Donna doesn't know what I'm going through]—
    Oh Nadine, I always feel a sense of well-being and focus after I talk with you! Did more in the last two hours than I'd done all day! lol
    Imagine yourself being a bird. A beautiful owl, perched high in the

tree. An owl is wise. And very instinctive. It could have been said to be a cardinal or eagle, but you will identify with an owl much more. Like many birds, an owl selects a certain spot to call home. She may have many temporary homes, or homes that she visits from time to time to fetch her food, but she will savor the sanctuary that her one particular home is. Did you know that an owl can turn her head right around to the back? She can look behind her in a second. She can look down from many tens of feet and see a tiny mouse running between the grasses on the ground. Within seconds, she can swoop down, gather the mouse up and nourish herself. She is very efficient and she lives in the Now. Now is the most important time for everyone. Everyone lives Now, everyone is born Now and everyone dies Now. Yesterday is nothing more than the remnants of Now and tomorrow is absolutely nothing more than Now on another day of the week. Essentially it's nonexistent. Because it has not yet come into creation.

All must live in the Now. All diseases and concerns are in the Now. Like the owl who does her hunting in the Now, your work can only be done in the Now. Now... is the most important time of all for everyone. When people take their energies away from the Now, and worry about past Nows and future Nows, they no longer have the ability to focus on the most important Now of all. It's funny that people worry about imaginary Nows, or Nows that don't even exist, or Nows that have evaporated to become nothing more than footprints washed away by oceans of life. Do not worry about anything except Now.

The owl that sits in the tree does not think about tomorrow, nor does she think about yesterday. She only thinks about Now, and the owl is said to be wise. If the owl needs to fly to another tree right Now, she flies. If an owl is happy sitting in her familiar tree Now, she sits. An owl never needs to worry about food, because there are many more mice running across the field than there are owls sitting in her tree. As people drive down the road and notice the owl sitting, perched in her tree, they gaze at her in awe. They take pictures of her, they talk about her to everyone they see shortly thereafter. A picture of her permanently rests in their mind. She becomes a real part of their Now. They don't realize it, but the owl has reaffirmed that there is beauty and grace in the world that is nothing of ordinary man's doing. It simply exists alongside of man.

You must be able to turn your head to see your back in a fraction of a second. You must be able to have vision beyond that imagined by others. You must have your instincts tuned into your perfect channel for perfect clarity. You must live only in the Now. If the owl was really to worry about the storm that sent branches on her tree flying and lingered on for days, she may be too distracted to gather her food Now. She does not think about yesterday. And if the owl was to expend her energies contemplating what the mice population may be tomorrow, she may miss the opportunity to gather what she needs today. That is why she only has one time. Now.

We are sending you what you must accomplish Now. We are sending you what you need to accomplish your tasks Now. We are behind you every step of the way Now. Old Nows and future Nows have no bearing on NOW. Now is where it's at, baby! Just worry about Now and use your energies, just like that owl. People ask you many times about their future Nows and that is funny. Their future Nows depend totally upon the energy that they contribute to that particular Now and we don't even know what they are going to do. However, we can give a good wager based on the ways they have managed their own Now energy. All people can change their growth by putting all of their energies into their Now and every day is a brand new Now. Well, you ask, how can that be, because if I didn't get groceries yesterday, I cannot eat Now. So, yesterday must matter, because it is causing my Now to be hungry. Let this be understood. Our Nows are lived in the footprints of Nows gone by. If the footprint is deep, or muddy, it may take the oceans of time longer to wash away its affects. But, if we were truly living in the Now, like the owl, we would be concentrating on what we need Now and our fridge would not be empty Now.

Regardless of the yesterdays, tossing away any thoughts of a tomorrow, life is Now, as it will always be.

We share our love with you, Nadine, and guide you to live in the most supreme time of all. NOW.

Gabrielle et al

At this point I was taking on too much responsibility to handle on my own. My body was vibrating out of control at night and it was hard to sleep. *Restless* was an understatement.

From Donna—

Hi Nadine, Wow – talk about vibrating beyond the normal realm of vibrations! lol It was great to see you last night and, to be honest, I don't know how you're keeping it all together.

You've got some big hurdles to jump, to move on to where you have to go. Those hurdles are in the Earthly plane, physical level and are very manmade. It's a huge challenge, to separate the Earth from the spirit as far as energy when there are so many souls reaching out to you. You are being bombarded, as others are drawing their connected souls towards you as well as you attracting your own. You must file. You have to return to the basics of your gifts.

Yes, people lie, people say things that they want brought to fruition, people do strange things, but they are simply living. They are simply people. Your talents of healing, your ability to open to the energies that are sent, may seem overwhelming, kind of like the doctor who opens his doors in the morning without any form of receptionist to make order in his day. You become bombarded and fragmented, which leaves you vulnerable. Chill.

You are attractive and in desire of companionship, and many would like to provide you with companionship, but you are in a transition period of growth, and how can you build on something when you are not finished building yourself?

People are of all different levels, and everyone wants to be on the best level possible. These are fragmented times. lol And there's a sense of amusement that so many people have now materialized to you that are wearing 'enlightened' clothing. They cannot enlighten themselves, let alone anyone else. lol

Enlightenment was meant to be used for people to connect to their higher selves – and that is us. lol Not for people to claim to have power over others. Or for people to pick up this and that of other people to manipulate a situation. They will pull in as much garbage as good, and dealing with the garbage of the wandering souls is not great. Wandering souls, you ask? Those are the souls that have some form of tunnel vision, and only see a connection with a higher vibration as something that will bring them material gain. As soon as they have what they want, whether it be a healing of body or heart, they are back to their own silly ways, creating the havoc that caused the issues to begin with.

It's been an experience for you, and you will decide as to the correct path that you must take. You cannot be responsible for the woes of others. You have your own woes which you must work around. Everyone has the ability to walk in one door and out the other if they so desire, and remember it's their life lessons, you do not have the ability to interfere with that.

Money will be a struggle for you, but within the next six months, you will be able to get a better grip on the situation. Government does not have a soul. Your life in selling real estate and other types of sales can be minimum in time and extremely lucrative and can provide you with a form of stability without fear – this avenue as a source of revenue has been given to you. It's not expected that you jump off of the ship's bridge and swim without a lifejacket 20 miles to shore. Use your manmade brain and make sure you do not suffer financially, because it has been given to you. Chill some more.

You must have a transition. Yes, you can sell your house if necessary, but it is not necessary. Focus on what you have to focus on, when you have to focus on it.

MEN… this is problematic. Yes, they want a physical romp. And you want an emotional connection. They'll give you an emotional connection with promises if you'll give them a physical romp. That is the way men are. You give them many gifts in ways that they don't understand, because it's just your nature. But they cannot bottle you up and take you home, and drink you whenever they want. They want you for different reasons, however, the main reason is that as they get older, the selection gets oh so slim. lol And you're pretty darn nice to have dangling off of their arm. You don't want to be a trinket, do you?

And face it: isn't having a lovely, shapely blonde to wake up to delightful for any man? Shake it off and don't be insulted at their needy nature. It's just the way that many are.

Turn off your phone, stop communications with all for 24 hours each week. Shut down your brain and meditate with us. We want you to rest. You are all messed up and you need to get rewired to move on. You're being bombarded by emotions and energies and we'd need 2 million pages to explain it all. It's not fun for you and it's not good. It was desired that you become a business woman of sorts with soul/physical healing in mind, but you haven't been able to put it all together because of outside influences.

This whole enlightenment thing is getting hilarious because everyone is apparently becoming enlightened – we don't know how. Enlightenment is an understanding that people are simply the physical forms which energy occupies. And love, peace, understanding and compassion are the components, yet a lot of yoyo's claim enlightenment when they are drawn to greed, lust and selfishness. That is what they manifest. Greed and lust and if they can get their fill by claiming some form of goodness, then that is the course they take. Happiness is a combination of having enough money to live on and doing what our purpose in life is. Not everyone has the purpose of being a fantastic person. Some have decided to come down to the Earthly plane just to be a greedy bastard. To change their life purpose mid-stroke is impossible.

Try to rest, Nadine, and pull your energies together. It is a lot of stimuli for you, but you have help when you need it. You're here to heal the few that can be healed, not save all the world.

Catch you later, Gabrielle et al

CHAPTER 10

Onward

My mission is to provoke you, to inspire you.

I felt I should write this book for those who are struggling to find the truth, to connect the dots to believe in their own destiny, for their higher purpose for the good of all.

The energy comes in 2 forms:

1. MIND – your thoughts are things and manifest amongst us, and

2. HEART – love vibrations.

Vibrations have rhythms. Involuntary rhythms can be transferred. We unconsciously compete for energy with those around us.

Mother Earth is speeding up faster than the human body can cope, forcing us through social chaos and environmental shifts in the Earth, to be conscious of what we want for ourselves. We can live in a hostile environment within ourselves or a positive one.

All of us are born with a spark that is easy to find again. That spark can help us see the truth. Enlightenment will help us get ready for the Earth's great changes. Enlightenment is the goddess awakening us up to help prepare for the Earth's new dimensions. New conscious awarenesses....

There are those that are born with special energies to purify soil, animals and plants. These people have high energies and naturally, even without thought, can purify. One of them is me. I have been chosen to teach, help and heal others as they come to the path. Apparently I agreed to this assignment before I was born.

Everyone on this planet is going through their own awakenings and enlightenments. We all are part of the vaccination to heal the Earth on some level. Discovering a dormant illness before it gets worse, touching nervous systems and unblocking energies are within the reach of all of us.

It has been said by many visionaries that the Mother Earth is talking to us by showing many catastrophies. These natural events are awakening us ALL so that we can purify the Earth. Scientists have been studying the alarming increase of cancer patients. More and more are being exposed to radiation around the world. This leads to the natural question of what we are doing to our food sources. Did you know we aren't getting the same nutritional value food had prior to World War I? We need to eat 40 pears today in one sitting to get the same nutritional value people got from one pear prior to the contamination of our food supply brought on by forced production. We need to think about balance to maintain healthy bodies.

How can we protect ourselves now to prepare?

Find your presence. Fill yourself up with warm and loving compassion. For me the best way to meditate and enter into contact with the light was by knitting. My Grandmother taught me that through repetition and harmony we learn to creatively visualize the power of intent. I could now be lost in my own world without being a victim. Most of us are not meant for solitude, and we only know ourselves when we see ourselves in the eyes of others. By finding your *I-am* presence, you increase your velocity and in return your dimension as the Earth prepares for its increase to the 5th dimension.

Awaken the repressed energy inside when you feel that push-pull feeling. For example, walk down the street and say, "I'm *here* and *now*."

Sit for a few minutes each day and do nothing, getting as much out of that time as you can, just *being*.

~ ✣

28 April 08, from Donna—

Good Morning, Nadine! I feel very warm and fuzzy inside being able to assist you on your journey.

Having a *calling* is such a strange thing to so many people. Perhaps a calling really stems from an agreement we made long before we cried our first tears on this physical plane? It's like the programming chip that we come with. What I find to be strange about a calling is the amount of resistance that our calling gets. Both from us and from those around us. I think it's difficult to fulfill some of these commitments because of the physical limitations we put on ourselves.

It's as though we know what our calling is, but once we start to taste the wine of the Earth, we are willing to delay our callings. Very interesting: we never seem to want to leave the party! lol Then we say things like: 'gee, if it was meant to be, it would be,' or 'if it is to be, I will receive the means to accomplish it.'

You have done the right thing. It's all about finishing. We can start a million things, have a million thoughts, but it's only the ones that actually get stamped 'finished' that are important. Imagine what a city would look like if no one had brought their thoughts to completion? Absolutely everything on this plane is the result of a thought, and the finishing of that thought.

It's like we have to be extra hard on ourselves. Say it, do it.

Dave, the guy of great dumpings, always stood in awe of completions. Like an alien life form on this planet saying, 'Look what this person did. Look what that person did.' Never realizing that there is no difference between that person and him, you or me. We are all capable of completing a task of greatness.

Your book – why is it important? It's important because you have in-

sight. Some people may deem it to be absolutely ridiculous. Some people may view it as the most important thing that they've ever read. Doesn't matter if it's a Jack and Jill picture book. What matters is that you set a deadline for completion, write it within that deadline, and bring it to life. Get it done.

Make it small. Make it easy. Make it a pocketbook that is simple to read and cheap to buy. An online e-book. Allow it to be a prelude for something more. You must simply finish it with ease. And when you do this, you will feel a sense of accomplishment and a power within yourself that you can in fact do this.

There are many avenues for your work: mini workshops, courses, self-help centers, many things, but don't focus on any of those right now. Just keep them as thoughts to yourself.

Keep your wishes quiet. You do not have the energies to battle off the nay-sayers. Do not say, 'I'm going to do this, I'm going to do that.' Simply do it. In broadcasting your intentions to the masses, you are opening yourself up to more negative energies than you can ever imagine. Besides, you are giving away your ideas, to be misconstrued and prostituted.

There are at least three real estate transactions that are sitting right in front of you which will come to completion within the next two weeks. You can bring them to you in a period of 72 hours if you focus on them right now. You are fragmented, and you are not understanding the complexity of the situation. Gee whiz, Nadine, you of all people should not be here for tutoring.

OK, focus on the course of least resistance. You have said you have it together right now, but we know different, and you must run yourself like a business. Money in… money out. You are not a genius who can write masterpieces on two hours of sleep a night, while living in a tent. Earn a good chunk of money via real estate sales, but take at least two days off a week to heal and one day off a week to write and one day a week to work on other business endeavors. This is by far the easiest route for you to take. Why is real estate the easiest? Because you know what you're doing and people are drawn to you. Get on a payment plan for taxes you will owe, and view yourself as a person capable of conquering all. Be careful about the time you spend away from home base right now, because you are a bit fractured, and it's easy for these things to come to you, rather than you go to look for them. They will find you. Think of us as your business manager. You need one… lol

Focus. Skip the date with the loser to write your plan. You have to put yourself into a different space of thought and time. Conserve your energies. Please do not broadcast your intentions, because it will serve as a negative towards your effort. Get this little book of soul literature done, without a lot of fanfare. A little owner's manual. Get it printed, then say, 'Hey, look at what I have just DONE.' That way, there is no negative energy towards your efforts. Just do it.

Website technology is a great idea. It is forever changing. Just keep focused and keep it simple. Perhaps now is not the time to think about intertwining real estate with spiritual teaching – we think it is not a great idea. However, you could touch on it. Seminars are a great way of reaching the masses. Your real estate money is at your back door. Not across the country.

So, you have said via a note to Donna that things are getting together. And we know they are, and the things we tell Donna to tell you are things that we are telling you directly but for some reason you feel more validity when they are in print from Donna. lol

Remember: nothing is worse than a good thought, a good intention that does not come to fruition, because it is energy tossed into the garbage can, and wasted. Cut the fat and zip your lips. Just get one small step done, completed, at a time. Tell people you cannot do something until you get another project done. Plan your week to include earning money, healing and working on a project. You cannot move ahead until you have straightened up with bodies of influence such as governments. So, make a schedule to get that straight. Plan out how many earning units you need to pay your debts. Budget wisely, and your goal will be reached painlessly and effortlessly. You just need to put your mind there and get the job done. Once you get this done, you will never be there again. For it will be done, and you can continue on your path with success. You cannot go through a new door until you are completely through the old door. You must shed some baggage.

Think high and strong. The strength and wisdom of our collective energies are with you.

Gabrielle et al

MUSIC TRACK
Everyone singing with Sara Bareilles in 'Love Song'
I learned the hard way
That they all say things you want to hear
And my heavy heart sinks deep down under you and
Your twisted words.

CHAPTER 11

Baby baby baby

April 29 08, journal entry
For all the lonely people...

Taking a break from writing this book, I go to my cell phone (being distracted? or led to in a mystical way? there are no coincidences) to retrieve a message from my Mr. For Now, Mike.

He says, "Sorry, baby, for not calling you back as I was at my mother's for two days."

I can't breathe. Bad vibes. Was it what he said this time? Going within, my instinct says he's not being honest. Didn't we just have this conversation between him and I? He knows my mind is insightful (that's why he said he was attracted to me). WHAT'S HE THINKING!?! besides knowing that I *know* about where he really was. Didn't his last message say two days ago that he left his mother's to go somewhere else? (He had to check in to tell me that, as he thought he was being nice and was deflecting where he was really going.)

Would it not matter if Mr. For Now wasn't physic himself and could sense another male figure hovering around me? Yup, his spider senses were tingling and he had to call three times in two hours to catch me on something he thought I was doing to be unfaithful (when I wasn't).

His fears in himself were signs for me. You bet my spidey senses were tingly.

Our history: I sensed Mike was having an affair with a married women and asked one of my insightful friends if he was flying someone in after me. Another women. They said no. Go and have a good time in Hawaii with Mr. For Now. Doesn't he bring in his birthday cards from his party two days ago signed and inked in lipstick. *Thanks for a great time and spending Christmas vacation with me.* Naturally I called him on it!

I like this guy – am I suppose to teach him something? What's he teaching me? Do I politely have a good time and then call it quits when I get back home? My physical body goes into fetal position. Tears of woe is me. Throw myself back to yesterday's terrible hurt and fears of men gone by. How is this guy going to handle me? I normally would hold it inside and try to fix them (the healer inside) and carry on. This time was different: it's gotten easier to tell my truth.

He admitted that he needed to 'close some doors' when he got home and promised me he would. Baby baby baby. Didn't I get a phone call with affirmation for me (and perhaps divine protection) that Mr. For Now flew in his *business partner* (which our *friends* didn't want anyone knowing) the very next morning after me!?! He called everyday from Hawaii to say he missed me so so much and he was all alone.

I called him on that one too and he said, "How can you be so smart?"

I could see her, tell you what she looked like, how many children she had, her birthday, etc.

He said, "You're right. I was wrong. Baby baby baby."

What to do? I have to be honest about my feelings. I called him thinking if he is in my life, I am to be his teacher. I could be very clear and *kind* and leave a message (because I would be empowered in myself to tell the truth, enlightened so to speak) and if he elected to learn from me he could be honest with himself and we could both move forward either way. Didn't this guy give me a song and dance about he was the first and only guy that loved me for who I was and appreciated me for being me? Didn't he say sorry for the last time he got by me?

If I got him on the phone, would he be like the rest and say, *Baby...*

baby… baby? (Those darn blank spaces between the dots seem to be getting longer.) Is this an archetype thing with men? Hey, back in the cavemen days, men couldn't go hunting unless they got a little lovin' from their women. Are things still the same except the lingo has changes from a *grunt grunt grunt* to *BABY BABY BABY?* Can't they be alone for one minute of silence and not run from one women to the next? Where's the discipline? Where's the respect for themselves? How would they feel if the tables were turned? Where's the consideration? Tunnel vision! Pure lack of vision, that's for sure!

I'm used to the twisted words. And got used to reading between the lines and listening to the blank stares. Is it better to be alone than unhappy?

Sorry, guys, this one needs to go down on paper to give strength and conviction to those who need a little guidance from up above. For all men and women alike, if we are all looking for spiritual wisdom and freedom, to give love freely and truly love ourselves. Who's in denial to just be reduced to searching for love in every crevice in our lives, to only being players in the field? How sad and lonely, I thought.

Something wasn't right.

Something has never been right, it seemed at this very moment, reflecting on most of my relationships.

One of the biggest questions if people look to discredit my abilities is *if she is so smart, why is she divorced and still single?* This needs to be addressed!

Why is it I can't breathe at times? Are *they* forcing us to talk to them, to breathe, to call for help? Help from our guides and angels. Are we just physical bodies that are guided by spirit and by fearing? Allowing people to come into my life to learn to overcome my thoughts that are driving my ego? What am I aspiring to? Why can't I just be happy being in the moment everyday… all day? Why do I need more?

Gabrielle, why do I seem to attract the same experiences when I know the lesson? Why do I have to have it repeated and repeated so many times? Follow my heart, you say. That's where I just don't get it – other than I am human too.

Why am I attracting the same type of men in my life?

A song typically plays over and over in my head, complete with

words and melody, to give me clues and messages that I need to pay
attention to, just at that very moment. Sometimes songs will come in
before I realize that I need direction. How clever (don't want to play
against me on *Name That Tune*). *Jumping jack flash, she's a gas gas gas.*
lol

Singing for me is therapy. They say your angels love it when you
sing and they bring you happiness and joy in return. This time a force
was making me sing over and over *Love Song* by Sara Bareilles.

Jump into my car. Drive to the nearest Future Shop to buy it. Guess
what's playing in the background – *Love Song*. No kidding! Jump in
the car. Rip open the wrapper, windows down, hair blowin', cool glasses on, singing in the mirror, checking my ego. *lol* The music is blaring:
*If all you have is leaving I'm going to need a better reason to write you a
love song today.*

Huh. I can breathe to think clear that I've come to this end of the
dating pool to realize a lot. The questions that run through your mind:
am I not meant to settle down? Why do I always attract men who can't
commit? Maybe I'm the one who doesn't want to settle down. Maybe
I just can't (not knowing fully what will happen – where my feet will
land). Maybe I get to grow up and be a big girl now?

Maybe if they are controlling, are they controlling out of their own
egos and fear? Is there such things as control? There is no such thing
as control! Where does karma play into those lives who try to control
you? (Oohh, that was my *outside* voice. I've got an 11-second rule. It's
like dropping gum on a sidewalk: you get to retrieve it and put it back
in your mouth. I took that comment back.) *lol*

If we are powerful reflective mirrors to one another, why do I attract
the most dangerous sorts? Is this good vs. evil? *Mirror, mirror, on the
wall. Who's the fairest one of all?*

They all were of the James Bond type. Soft quiet type at first. Looking
for their next adventure and silently carrying a gun, dressed to kill.

They came in all packages: tall, short, full head of hair to no hair,
green, blue, brown eyes. There were Porches, Ferraris, Cadillacs,
Audis, to pick-up trucks to the average sedan. These were considered

to me all relationships and whom I all cared deeply about (I was what
I thought to be fully loyal and committed). Truly! Please bless all their
hearts!

There was a similar theme. The danger, the excitement, they intrigued my mind to learn more from them. The conversations were
deep over red wine and the odd cigar! I could think like a guy!

～❧～

30 April 08, journal entry—

I'm realizing all the discussions and telephone calls weren't enough
to set my boundaries. Some of these guys just don't know when to
quit.

I just wrote this standard letter for ending relationships. I can quickly fill in two blanks for *To* and *From*. Who would possibly come back
for more after my letters!

|Imagine this a tear-out page for anyone who has been in an un-
healthy relationship, to make it easy and to give purpose and a fresh
start to someone's life.| I think people need direction to help them with
the next step when all else fails. Boundaries give hope and promise.
Pruning is GOOD!

Dear _____ ,

I am taking responsibility for the situation that was presented to me
by you, and by me to you. I want to build some comfort that I dealt
with this matter as best as I could for you, as you will be in other situations that come your way. Below you will see conversations of the truth.
Thought you should know – again I apologized to you that it has come
to this.

Missing you terribly, but you ripped my heart wide open yet again,
this time for the last time.

We've had conversations in the past and I felt you were making me
out to be this terrible person and unfit for you. I was always willing to
work through your situations but you have no time left for me. Love
is patient and love is kind. I have been in this situation seeing the same
patterns – me being patient, waiting for you over a period of time, to

be yet again blamed for you not being strong enough to transition to what you manifested. Blamed for being me and what I can teach you. What did I reflect to you? What do you see about yourself? Let's be honest and both apologize. We learned. We brought truth even if we don't agree.

Problem: there is so little time left between us to discuss issues it is imperative to resolve. There was no resolve to build trust. Nothing has changed. Let's surrender, that's the easiest way to go through life and the most rewarding. Ego versus spirit. So much to learn to go through life, and it's that much easier when you surrender to spirit and let go of the control. Things are what they are. Let go of the control, live in the spirit and love, just love and trust that we are not meant to be together at this time. I wish you all the happiness and joy, and want you to share that with someone who cares, believes and will respect you. It's not an equal relationship. I want more than you can give me.

I was the light, the dream, and the energy and spirit you aspired for, yet the fog and drama between us blocks you so that you aren't crisp to see. If you could let go of fear and prune the ego, you would be free and everyone around you would feel the love. There is no one else that understands that more than I do at this time, and there's so much more you needed to see and learn. In the process I have been deceived terribly and hurt so that I can't continue to respect you. Everything is as it should be. Please find more acceptance as I have learned from you, thank you for being my teacher, respect your level of awareness and wish you happiness in your journey.

So that there is no misunderstanding, I loved you completely and was always there waiting for you, even when I knew so much more at my expense. I only wished we could have gone through life together to share each other's dreams.

Compassion, love and respecting you,

(signed) _____

The ultra-rich Prince Harming can't literally climb into my head, but he can telepathically interfere with me day and night. We separated well over six months ago. Even when you say goodbye, is it goodbye? This one wasn't like the rest. He had powers too. Powers to *telepathically speak*. Powers to have a relationship on another plane perhaps? Another new learning experience for me.

His energy can attach to me. I can actually feel his heaviness, the burdens he put on himself through his thoughts. Why me? Why do I get his pain? I learned to send him love from a distance. My pain then would go away. There was no mistake that he was thinking of me and attached to my energy field. I had to learn to repair that protective boundary around me, so that he couldn't harm me anymore.

While we were together it was uniquely bonding. He would be awake and mentally try to wake me up (we lived in different cities). He did this out of a dead sleep (my phone was shut off). I would wake up, turned on the phone to receive his call within one minute. At the time, it was fun and exciting that we were that in tune with each other. Now is a different story: we aren't together and I am trying to move on with my life.

A heaviness comes over me and, recognizing that feeling, it's as if the pressure in my chest wants me to get the energy out on paper or repeat the message that is being received. I never know when these messages will come in. Sometimes when I am most relaxed (watching TV, at the movie theater, at dinner).

Fatila brava [meaning *do what is right and kiss me* in Italian] was ringing in my ear.

Once more. [It was him. ugh.]

Goodbye, my sweets, time to go. Say good-bye to your daddy in charge. Let me see, you found someone else? [He was being sarcastic. The messages were mixed as his mind was too; up and down were his thoughts.]

Larceny at best. Diamond ring store nearby. Gateway to heaven, you are for me. Practice makes perfect. Baby, in charge no more? Found a place in my heart forever, diamond bracelet won't do, diamond necklace won't do, heart-shaped pendant won't do, what to do? [This guy was worth millions and tried to play that card with me. He couldn't understand why that wasn't going to work with this woman.]

Tired of the same old wenchless past?

You need me, I know, feel your pain.

Heartaches, heart strings. Carry on without me – a must to simplify your life.

Boys will be okay without me.

Hard to say goodbye, but a must I feel. You need attention of the heart. Lunge at me like no other.

Mystic ways no more with me.

Hard to acknowledge the truth – how do I do that, how do I start? Paring order in place. I need space to figure things out no more.

Want you back. Want you next to me. Come here.

Go away, thoughts.

Breathing the air you do.

For me it's easy to say goodbye, you need me when...

|Angels said:| *No go, Ms Mercey. Trapped in society, can't get out. Double up income no more. Heartache.*

Heart break, you mean.

Captivated by your heart. One more day, one more dollar.

A friend told me the truth about you. Trapped in society, can't get out.

Captivated by your heart.

One day at a time. Practice makes perfect.

We make a perfect pair.

Dumb blonde, why did I wait to tell you?

She will dance no more for me, I want you. Placing a bet that you will marry me in the end if I ask you.

Cry on my shoulder. |It's a form of reconciliation, if you must, not entirely what he had in mind.|

Dumb blonde brunette not worth my time in gold.

You are needing help.

Pray for me. That's all I ask. Can't say why I did it. Needed company.

Past is past. Let's move forward.

Necessary measures must be taken into account – the fact that you are gorgeous stop traffic if required.

Dumb blonde, why did I regret last reconciliation?

Stems of affection for you. Pure diehard sheep, skin black night, watch maiden journey.

This life is no more for me. Hard to let go.

Most of my past with her. Tried to tell her nicely. Won't let go.

No.

Yes… |went his thoughts.|

- ❦

Angels speak to me now—

He's back. No, not entirely – wants you to believe he will, to keep you on the line. Heartache at best.

Stay away, Ms Mercey!!!!

Do not be wishing things were different. Wishing things were done with ex aren't naïve at best on your part, Ms Mercey. Needed a shake up in the head. Yesterday we relieved you of the grief you were about to endure. Heart attack on a plate that man is. Ready to explode to New York and back. Had an affair naïvely on your part. Take a hold of what you know and use it to your advantage not to spite the man but believe you have been rescued from up above. Trapped in a man's space of hope for survival. That's all, nothing more, nothing less.

Helped you from afar. Now help us. Let us give peace to the rest of the society at large by telling your story. Keep it fair, keep it light. Have a heart and give peace to the rest of the liars out there. Won't be theirs to lose, yours to gain in every angle of deceit, lies and deception. Forwarding a plan as we speak. Kept quiet, kept captive in your own peace of mind and anguish.

Why did you let a man like that speed your love to us; you needed revenge on the other? Perhaps, maybe not. You're in charge, you're in control. Have a heart for the wicked and lonely. Have a heart for the peace that is about to shake you free from the anguish and deceit that was pressed upon your chest so tight previously. Stepping up to the plate as we speak.

Kept captive by the design and form of his father and mother before him. Have a heart for the weak and needy. Have a heart for the lonely and departed. Have a heart, for the record player will play your song.

Have a heart for the decapitated body before you have a heart for the iron-clad man in stone is back, back in the saddle again he feels. No more for the man of greed, kept it quiet, kept it clean for a while until you were. Grieving you, your loss of the man of steel. Freeze frame, take a picture for what it is: deceit, entrapment, if you let it. Dializes his wishes, free man now. Locked up and thrown away the key!!!

Prince Harming is back in my mind—

Past is past. Let's move forward, love, please. Have a favor, will you marry me? Diamond proposal at best from the starts, from the wishes you held dear.

Teach me again. Speed your love to me. Heartache, heart break. Stop me from drowning. Nerve racket. Nerve endings. Near me, I am lost without you. Can't breathe. Can't eat. Can't dine without you. Nerve endings, nerve heart break. Can't take another day without you, must see you. Please.

Angels again—

Faith at hand, take charge of your life. Kids more important than lies and deceit, will get you nowhere fast if you take that route. Over and out, my dear. Saved. Outraged at last. He teaches himself a lesson. Hard core no more. Hardache at best. Stepping up to the plate. Needs space no more. Wants lessons in reverse.

[Whew. I was being protected again. Now they were close at hand, showing me how to block his mind-speak.]

Are our thoughts our reality?

Was I being warned not to give airspace or breathe an ounce of energy to this competition for energy? Yes. Would I repeat these patterns again? Would the lesson for me get louder if I wished him back? I was saved by my angels this time, but was I learning a lesson?

I was certainly trying to!

This wealthy man wanted me to wait water and feed him at his beck and call when he wanted me. Put me on a shelf – when he wanted to pull me off, I needed to be available. He liked having women on his arm for show (I'd once thought I was the only one). "Baby baby baby, I look after you," he'd said. "You have no worries."

MUSIC TRACK
Whitesnake performing 'Here I Go Again'
I don't know where I'm going
But, I sure know where I've been
... Made up my mind
I ain't wasting no more time.

CHAPTER 12

Forward and westward

Let's wind our story back to 2007 to properly introduce this...
The Universe responds quickly when you're on the right path.

It took me three hours to get ready, to put the suit on that morning. How much more makeup or hair gel could I apply? My physical body just didn't want to go to the office.

I went and, without a plan or thought, I found myself taking down the awards and plaques. I was a successful veteran in the business. People were staring. What are you doing? I'm done. Tears rolled in joy, not knowing what next step I would take or how I would get there. I just knew I was done. The switch turned off.

Within two weeks after severing all ties with that office and becoming fully broke and fully independent, new doors opened quickly. I committed to edge my way out of real estate and become a full-time healer. Couldn't afford a boutique office, so I began healing from a room at home.

For 20 years I sold real estate. How do you start a new business with no money, no web site, no advertising? Yet I was soon booked weeks in advance.

Initially my hourly rate was less than half that charged by healers with my talent. This worked to build testimonials and referrals quickly. People were being treated. Testimonials flowed in. Presents. Thank-you cards. It was my affirmation that this was the rewarding career I had been waiting for.

Automatic writings were coming in directly from my angels again! This time something about *martial arts expert required for Prince Harming; Angelina Jolie, Brad Pitt, Hotel California*. Hmmm. How could anything involving Brad Pitt be bad? *lol*

Two months later, as I was healing a client in my home, I got a very profound internal message to go to my former realty office immediately after the session. I did. Went to the mail box to see only one piece of paper.

I'd trained my body to give me a sign. My body talked to me (or talked back to me it seemed) when I needed direction. I got a shot of electricity or goosebumps (God bumps, so to speak) when I saw this advertising flyer from Good Life Fitness. I hadn't heard of this company before and wasn't aware what was to come, but I knew this was a dot that must be connected somewhere.

My girlfriend Paula was very protective of me. She had the gift to channel for my protection when I needed her. Paula told me I *should* go out that night. Not remembering that she guided me and being human with doubts and fear, I told her I didn't want to go out into the social scene. She argued with me and pushed me hard to go out to a specific place.

I did.

A man from across the room came over (I read him and knew he was looking at my unusual aura). He said his name was Mike and asked what I did for a living. Normally I would say real estate agent. Mike was special too I felt – with gifts to see, feel and hear energy. I told him I was a healer.

He asked me to do a few parlor tricks as some do when in doubt (which is good, it gives pause and reason to believe). Another person to open, I thought.

We became more relaxed talking about my healing abilities. He said he had some magic of his own too! (Girls, this was not a line. *lol* Or was it? blonde. dumb. *lol*)

I asked him where he lived (we were in Hamilton, Ontario). He said Vancouver and he was only here for the day and was on business for Good Life Fitness!

Goooooossseeebbbuummppss… another dot connected.

I asked him, "You aren't a martial arts expert, are you?"

He said yes. He was going to California and was working with Warner Brothers and would be on set with Angelina Jolie and Clint Eastwood. Another dot. Space between the lines.

I said I wasn't interested in dating (at all). He *knew* our meeting was important as he had received an internal message that I needed to go to LA [Los Angeles] to find out who I was. Mike would teach me that healers in the phone book on the west coast (unlike Ontario) are like Smith in a phone book.

I was excited with this news. I wasn't born on the hippy dippy coast, didn't have an ethnic, spiritual person on each side of me growing up. Heck, my Mom and Dad didn't know what to make of me – they thought my vibrations and headaches meant I was allergic to chocolate. I had talked to very few people about my abilities. As Mike talked, I was becoming comfortable that someone wanted to open doors and show me the way.

This guy had stories. Besides training Clint Eastwood, Mike had also worked with Sylvester Stallone, Chuck Norris, Steven Seagal, Hilary Swank, the list goes on.

He said he needed spiritual coaching and paid me up front for several healings. We talked and struck a friendship and certain respect for one another. Our paths had collided in an unconscious universal exchange of energy. An unanticipated journey was just beginning in my career.

Two weeks later, I'm in California with Mike. We were invited to go on set of a new film at Universal Studios with Angelina and John Malkovich as Clint's guests. We shopped for Angelina's and Clint's gym equipment but didn't make it to the set in time due to LA traffic.

Mike had met Angelina and described her as someone with a definite presence of power. We didn't meet her this trip.

I remember getting a coffee and the attendant asked when I was going back to Canada. He didn't know me or where I was from and this is how Californians start a conversation! Spooky. I was taken aback, thinking he was reading me, then wondered if he'd simply picked up on my Canadian accent. He then continued, "You're a powerful healer, huh?"

Now I was *spoooooooked*. I said, "How did you know?"

He said, "I felt what you just did to me."

I wasn't trying to transmit energy. My energy sometimes automatically transitions to people without my knowledge. Sometimes I realize this as my breathing or voice changes. But the recipients generally don't know, depending on their velocity level.

Mike's friend brought a date to dinner. She asked what I did for a living. I looked over at Mike to ask if it was okay, not sure if he was getting used to me being a healer and wondering how would people react. He nodded so I told the lady, and she gave my name to someone she met in a bar the next evening. By the time I got back to Canada there was a phone message to call LA: a new client. He needed help desperately. There was hope that I would help him from a distance. I began sending energy. I could feel we were improving his memory. Within days, he was getting better. His wife Lilly wanted to fly me back to LA in three weeks to do more healing and to meet me in person to discuss his situation.

She offered to pay for the full expense of flight, car, hotel, food, phone. I accepted, a bit uneasily because I wasn't used to people paying my way. I emailed Lilly a few testimonials, which she immediately emailed and passed on to friends, some in the media. People called to book appointments. She was getting her nails done in Beverly Hills, told the manicurist, who told another influential lady we'll call K.

I received a phone call from K the next day and sent energy from a distance. She felt the shift instantly. Did a reading for her. Struck up an instant relationship. K wanted to meet me when I landed in LA. I trusted her... but I didn't know who she was.

I got to LA and started back-to-back healings – networking had brought in many needing help. Lilly could see auras and knew her husband's energy was clearing and she could see an improvement in his functioning at that time.

K lived in the hills of 90210. She lived at the very top. I got out of the car and hugged her as if I had known her from before, because it certainly felt that way. We jelled. K asked me to stay in the guest house to help save Lilly some money. Monogrammed linens, fresh flowers, silver water canteen by my bed. Upholstered walls, pictures of presidents Nixon, Carter, Clinton, Reagan with her husband. He had been a federal undersecretary of state.

Me, a small town girl from Brantford who's never been to California, just had to ask K (the finest debutant hostess) to tell me some famous celeb stories. She had some reluctance because, as she expressed it, she wanted me to be *pure* for my healings. "Nadi, please don't change," K said.

She'd made dinner for Mrs. Bush, had danced with Cary Grant, Ava Astaire was in her dance class (Fred would come and watch his daughter dance), Candice Bergen was a close friend, her brother hung out with Jack Nicholson. The stories and names would go on.

I found K to be extraordinarily grounded and appreciative of my company. She had traveled the healing circuit and said she checked me out through other intuitives around the world to see the power of this energy, and if I was pure or not. Did I pass the test? Well, I could read in her mind what other readers were saying to her – I passed the test.

We toured the city. She showed me where her Grandma lived on famous Doheny Drive in a huge mansion! Theirs was a wealthy oil family. I'm starting to connect the dots from the past angel talk. Ferraris in the garage. Old antique cars. No, they are too grounded and nice to have all this, I thought. They must have earned it and respected the money along the way. Her husband tells a wonderful life story, almost a Forrest Gump in his own right. Retired from the highest levels of power in the Capitol, he now builds homes for the likes of Johnny Carson, Tom Cruise, Madonna and the Beanie Baby fellow Ty Warner. (I remember this dot with the beanie babies. *lol*)

I was looking after the dogs Jilly and Angus, wiping their paws on an old towel with the White House emblem on it – *lol* – as my hosts went to a debate at the Reagan Library with Mrs. Reagan. Arnold Schwarzenegger was two seats from them as I was watching on TV.

K was kind and had set up, without me knowing, some healing for some prestigious notable people from Beverly Hills in her living room. We were soon making a splash with the energy! Everyone loved the experiences.

One day as K was getting a work-out with her trainer, I sent her energy to boost her training. That was a first!

Daniel Lue was the first Asian on the hit TV show *Survivor*. When I met him, I realized another angel talk dot was connected.

Excellent trip. I was booked to come back next month, and the next, and the next. It was amazing how the connections happen so well – as if all this was meant to be!

The media/celebrity vibrations were sky high on my return trip to Canada. Now at the airport heading home, my trip was delayed. I was told to go to a service counter and reschedule my flight due to a snowstorm. I was given the last flight to Canada that night. My luck, or divine intervention?

Pat Boone was right in front of me at the security gate. Do you always bump into celebrities there? Or was it me?

On the plane I sit beside the wife of a former US Admiral of the Navy. They are retired and were telling me of their trip back from Australia, her daughters are pilots flying missions to bring doctors in to help children who are sick overseas. They were looking to find someone to put together a deal to bring Beanie Babies, stamped with the US Navy, as a token for the children there. Gggoooossbbuummmppss. Didn't I just stay with the man who is building Mr. Beanie Baby's house?!

That's me... Ms Forrest Gump. Life unfolding in an amazingly positive way.

Was she led to say that to me? Were K and her husband led to talk about Ty Warner to help these children, to give hope and bring love to their hearts? Are we all connected universally as part of this healing vaccination to help heal the people, which will heal the Earth?

Get this. I get off the plane for my connecting flight in Dallas. I find myself wandering and wandering and wandering around this small shop without buying anything. For some reason I am not moving. I notice my breathing start to get heavy. I'm hot as if I am clearing someone. There's only one other customer in the shop. Actor Owen Wilson is right behind me....

When the flight lands at the Toronto airport I felt compelled to buy *People* magazine. (I never buy *People* magazine.) At the newsstand, I locate a copy and who is on the front cover that month but Owen Wilson. All I knew was that, given my gift and talent, I wanted to help him and felt that I could. Maybe, just maybe, we exchanged energy. In fact I know we did – though he probably didn't know.

Was my flight delayed so I could get the last ticket on an alternate flight through Dallas, so I would bump into Owen? And bump into the retired admiral who needs to connect with the Beanie Baby man? Everything happens as it should. *lol*

When I got back to my home, there was a message to call Big Coat Productions. They wanted to see me in their office in Toronto. I googled them: they are a TV production company.

"Who wants to pick my brain now?" I thought.

This is the story on how Home & Garden TV found me. I went to a real estate refresher course in Toronto. The location was Paula's choice – she wanted to socialize afterwards. (I was debating at the time whether to keep my license current to sell real estate or not. One foot in, one foot out. It could be good back-up.)

The teacher asked me a question. I answered the question which led into a lengthy conversation about my recurring dream that became an awakening dream in a particular home. I was explaining my awareness that spirit can play havoc with energies in homes and cause disruptions to one's health and certainly cause damage to electrical circuits. I knew this from 20 years of experience selling real estate.

The teacher said, "Can you say this again for Home & Garden TV?"

Wwhhhaaa! Paula slapped me on the leg and said, "These things happen only to you, Mercey."

Yup. Producers interviewed me afterwards, and I was invited to film a pilot as the host for a TV show! *lol* All I could think of is what shoes should I wear.

Two days back from LA, the Universe was working overtime to make whatever opportunities and awareness I needed to teach happen very quickly.

The house that I went to for the pilot filming was an experience in itself. I had *no* prior knowledge of why or what I was there for.

I arrived. Late, of course. Walked into the home. Who's home?? And was instantly hit by a vibration so strong I couldn't breathe. This energy didn't want me there!

b... bb... b... bbreathe.

Just like the big black prisoner in the movie *The Green Mile,* who was wrongly accused and who cleared the little mouse and in turn the warden's wife of disease, I automatically take on energy and release it. Often in the form of a burp.

I was burping in the front hall, trying to be discrete about it. The crew asked me not to as a man was being filmed in the home apparently measuring paranormal energy with a machine.

I shut myself up in the room set aside for makeup, and had to clear that space... so that I could breathe.

A young man came in and asked if I was wearing a bra. Huh? Why would he ask that? Dumb blonde who has never filmed before – that was tech talk for do we need to buffer the material noise and rig the mic... MIC! Oh my god, they are going to mic me for appearing on camera.

Cameras everywhere. It was all quite shocking and overwhelming. What did they want me to do? What do I say?

An assistant came to get me and said, "Open the door and start doing your thing."

What *thing?* Everything in my life with energy and who I was wasn't a problem – others were controlling the energy and directing me, it seemed.

The angels were talking louder, and making me laugh. They wanted me to sing. I was laughing out loud. And started doing what they wanted me to do. Then more angels began interfering or someone was, so that I wasn't clear at first. I had to take charge. It worked. I was super, super clear and went into a natural mode and projected on camera exactly with the detail and phrases they were looking for. As if it were all channeled (get the pun?). The stars were aligned (yes, another pun)! No take-overs. It was smooth, fast and accurate.

We captured on film the speaking, the energy locations, hot spots so to speak, all confirming the results from the energy measuring machine.

It all boiled down to a laundry floor drain in a closet! Sppooookkky. That energy didn't want me there. I couldn't stand it and had to leave the immediate area of the basement. I cleared the energy from upstairs, and the angels made me sing and dance, *Talk to me, baby, nice and low* and *Ghosts in the material world.*

It was a take! The producers knew they had something – it was time to edit and go to market.

Word soon came that Vision TV was very interested in doing a documentary about my healing abilities. I hope they can figure out how to photograph auras and the feelings associated with each color. Love is pink. If a client wants more spiritual direction, in comes purple energy. For those who need to be grounded, a crimson color shows. Gold is higher than the typical white spirit connection.

Wonder what's next in this ever-entertaining world?

MUSIC TRACK
Listen to Erasure's 'Chains of Love'
How can I explain when there are few words I can choose
... when words get broken?

CHAPTER 13

Where is this leading?

May 2 08, journal entry—
[Dear Diary: as you might have predicted, Mike and I are becoming an *item*. This is a message I emailed to Mike—]

Transpire to think with your heart.

Pure love and light is what I reflect to you. I am what you repel when you can't just *be*, and love yourself. Different mind sets, different energies, different fabrics (even without speaking).

It's a beautiful thing to help others – be conscious of that! Life will do you better favors that way!

We can't come together unless you stop the stammer and do what you intend to! The intent could be there, but the full purpose isn't truly there yet.

If you don't have the answers and are standing still, that's a sign your mind can't function unless you bale out old habits and thought patterns. Close those doors of yesterday, don't choose to fight with the change. When you stray from your path, this causes stress and emotion and physical break down. Feel it. Know it when you're on top. You're on track! The Universe will respond quicker to your thoughts and desires.

I will help you when you want it, though you need to make the conscious choice first. Turn on the switch!

Still offering the knowledge, I see so clearly that *some people just don't want to change*. You might feel the emotional release but that's just the tip of the iceberg. You may get locked into or slip back to stay in the patterns that you think you've mastered, but I know you want to transpire for so much more life.

Look at the pictures. You made choices to be with your heart. Only you know that.

I will help you, but you have to work at it. *Every day.*

I'll wait for your affirmations. I will know the truth, for the light side is winning!

Acknowledge yourself and inspire yourself to get the best support around you as possible. You will need it. More emotion is on the way.

Much energy and love,

Nadine

5 May 08, journal entry—

Does God have a daytimer for us? Does he check his calendar and text message us for the next important meeting of the day?

I stopped wearing wrist watches and went with the flow. Actually my mindset changed when I purchased a bracelet watch for $10.00 that *always* read 11:59. How clever to work as if it's the last minute of the day. |Traded in my Gucci. Umm, uh, let me run up to my jewelry box to remember: Cartier or Movado? *lol* |

Soon I began to operate on the time that was given to me. I was more productive this way it seemed. Never have I been lost for words with this mindset while writing this book. I sat down today to write and the phone rang every hour on the hour – calls from three different people from all walks of life. They all had something to share, to teach me. Their calls reminded me to include them in my story. I hadn't heard from these people in months. How beautiful to hear from them, to hear how their journeys were growing. Drew called from New York – a world traveled healer/lecturer/networker and thrill seeker of the spirit world. Andrea is a blonde, dreadlocked, crystal street vendor from Venice Beach who I got talking to the first time I was in Cali. Vaughn is a famous bodybuilding veteran, old school street fighter, turned professional trainer. People just bump into your path when you need them. We can all help each other. In an exchange (because the Universe finds it important to exchange), you never know what one person can bring to the table, who they know, or what you can offer them.

My phone conversation was short due to a bad phone connection with Andrea on the beach. She'll call back. I know it's important, that little street vendor from the south. It's about connecting the dots. I know we can help each other.

Vaughn was delivering an exercise bike to my house, as a gift from someone I was healing. I did a healing for Vaughn as he had dislocated his shoulder, and introduced him to a product that could build his business. He is helping other people heal through this high antioxidant drink. Is it about the juice, the bike, the gym? It's about lending a hand, turning a good dead for those who need it, for those who care. You get to pay it forward! By increasing one person's velocity, you get to increase the world's.

I realized how lucky it is to have good people in my life to help influence others, to tell their story. They are all healers too. They just might not all know that. They are all part of this vaccination process to heal the world – as you are too! What I didn't realize is that they were in my daytimer on the list of things to do. Things to do and people to listen to, so that I may teach others.

***

Karyn Reece (TV psychic and medium for police detectives) asked me to lecture at her Psychic and Paranormal Expo in Getzville, NY last fall. I was speaking on *Thoughts are Things*. Drew Pearson was speaking on *Orbs*. As I was waiting for my lecture to start, Drew felt drawn to come out during his talk into the hallway and asked me to come join the group. Drew wanted me to send energy to the group of people [this was my first group energy session]. Frankly, I didn't know what orbs were but didn't want to admit how limited my vocabulary was. The lights were turned down to capture the energy glow by camera as I was working with the energy. Drew took a picture of the crowd. Orb energy appropriately landed on a gentleman's heart – it was amazing as that man had heart problems and needed the energy precisely at that time. Now I saw for my own eyes what orb energy was. I knew from my experience that I could bring it in and work with it in a healing capacity. This was getting interesting. It appeared to me that spontaneous healing brought in the healing spirit – *that's* what appears as a glow of light.

We can't *control* it. Speaking with Drew we agreed we were just pawns in that configuration. We were in the right space for that very moment. The Universe could care less if the human was ready or not.

Drew had the following to comment on orbs:

The term orb is the popular name first given in 1996 to typically circular anomalies appearing in photographs. In photography and video, orbs appear to be balls, diamonds, or smears of light with an apparent size ranging from a golf ball to a basketball. Orbs sometimes appear to be in motion, leaving a trail behind.

There are two main trains of thought regarding the cause of orbs in photographs. The first school sees it as a fairly clear-cut case of flash or sunlight reflection off of dust, particles, insects or moisture droplets in the air in front of the camera, i.e. they are naturalistic. The opposing school maintains that orbs are paranormal in nature, i.e. non-naturalistic and spirit-like.

Some people claim that paranormal orbs are more likely to appear in certain locales, or are attracted to human activities, especially those involving children. The images on Internet sites devoted to orbs are taken in graveyards, backyards, attics, kitchens, living rooms as well as cars, convention centers and city streets – in short, anywhere people may be taking photos. Locations in which orbs are frequently observed are often said to be associated with other supposedly supernatural activity and haunting taking place.

During my second visit to California I went out into the night on the famous Santa Monica Pier in my flip-flops in the cold January rain. I walked to the end of the pier in the dark night and breathed in the rich ocean air. I was led to take digital pictures. Orb energy appeared in all the pictures, something that has never happened before to me. Walking closer to the Ferris wheel, I had the intent in my mind to place orb energy on the spindles. I have the picture that shows my intent worked: placing energy strategically, and large amounts of it, all at the right time and with the right intention. Sure enough, it's there in the snapshot! Who would have thought – are we purposely being taught by these paranormal affirmations to fight against society's *normal* teachings? Hhhhmmmm.

⸙

Drew Pearson and I agreed there are three types of healings: verbal, physical and meta-physical.

Verbal healing is a form of mediumship. In a group discussion you can share information that flows to you, to raise awareness and help heal. For example, you can describe to the person what color (aura) they represent, what animal do they remind you of, what aspects of that animal do they form.

My sons Eric and Jaxon and I sit in the hot tub in the back yard and look up at the stars and talk. They love playing a game where Jaxon will think of an aura color linked to a particular feeling. I read him and take on that color and feeling. Eric will read my aura and describe it out loud. The very first time he did this, Jaxon burst out with amazed laughter. He recognized that you could think a color and learn what that color vibration felt like. Eric was matter-of-fact: "Yeah, so?" *lol*

[Note: playing this game was important. Jaxon as a 4-year-old saw apparitions or spirits. He was afraid one day after seeing one in his room, ran away and didn't return to his bedroom for weeks later. Jaxon chose to shut down his gift (at that time). This game gave Jaxon a method to be attached to the energy in a way that he was comfortable.]

Physical healing is the typical Reiki hands-on healing technique that is becoming acceptable in hospitals today as *Therapeutic Touch* [often called TT]. Usually the hands don't actually touch the person's skin, but hover above to sense where healing is needed and to move energy. Therapeutic Touch has been proven effective in clinical trials, so that it is now taught to nurses. This is a positive sign that the western medical establishment has now verified a healing method that has been practiced around the world for probably a million years, and is getting more comfortable with methods for which there is no mechanistic scientific explanation.

Meta-physical healing is using your mind to send energetic messages emanating from our positive and negative thought. This form of healing shows that genes and DNA do not control our biology; that instead DNA is controlled by signals from outside the cell, showing our bodies can change by the way you think.

It's certainly an interesting time being a healer. It should be accepted and understood that this is a widespread natural ability and *not* a special gift. I believe we are all born with profound intuition.

The greatest system of healing is sometimes referred to by scientists somewhat derisively as the *placebo* effect. Placebo is the Latin word for *I please*, and this refers to the spontaneous healing that can take place when the patient simply *believes* his or her condition will improve. For example, some patients given a dummy pill (called a placebo) will heal just as well or better than those given a pharmaceutical drug. Pharmaceutical companies tend to dismiss this natural healing process because it messes up their studies and drug trials, and they can't make any profit off mock pills and positive thinking. Medical doctors are put into a bind since they know the placebo effect is very common and can be more powerful than drugs, yet having a patient improve simply because of confidence in the doctor seems to put these 'men of science' in the same category as a faith healer or native shaman. Nevertheless, a recent study revealed that over half of all US doctors admitted to regularly prescribing placebos to patients. Surveys in Denmark, Israel, Britain, Sweden and New Zealand have found similar results.

There are a few organizations now undertaking critical research that is showing how, if your intent is strong enough, your body system will follow the quest and recover.

Gandhi said, "Be the change you want to see."

He meant social *and* personal changes. You have to heal yourself first to be a positive force in society.

"Many problems, essentially man-made problems... are created due to the demarcation of *we* and *they*. On that basis, the whole concept of war happens.

"World peace depends on the inner peace of individuals, which in turn comes from compassion and affection for others. Constant anger, jealously, agitation and fear are damaging to one's health and are a form of *suicide*.

"Whether you love others or not, your existence depends on them, that's a reality." — the Dalai Lama.

6 May 08, journal entry—

As a child thinking about what I would become, I didn't grow up wanting to be a healer or teacher of some sort. Hospitals, doctor's office – *ugh*. Working with people who were dying? Who were desperate for change? I was afraid of catching a cold!

I was a girly girl who played with Barbies, had every doll, Shirley Temple, Cher with her elaborate wardrobe – lived the girl fantasy of *Here's Barbie, Here's Ken*. Let's live happily ever after, drive off into the sunset in my powder blue Malibu Barbie convertible with the surf board in the back.

At 4 o'clock I would race home after school, put on my special *I Dream of Jeannie* pajamas and watch Barbara Eden and Larry Hagman. I was the genie. I was fixated on the dance as she came out of the bottle, then I sat cross-legged on the floor, arms precisely crossed, nodding my head to grant wishes. Sweet adorable, blonde and bubbly. That's who I wanted to be. To be the servant to my master. Kissing him on the cheek as he came home after a hard day at the office. *lol*

Samantha Stephens wasn't a bad witch, she was a good witch in the hit TV series *Bewitched*. I walked around my parents' home as a little girl, wiggling my nose. *lol* Did she influence me? "Try to control your temper. Remember peace on Earth and goodwill towards men includes witches too!" advised Samantha.

When it comes to Santa Claus, most mortals don't believe he exists.
Just like they don't believe in witches. I was not afraid of ghosts who
bumped into the night; it was the ice cream truck that scared me. To
this day when I hear the eerie, trance-like musical jingle of the ice cream
truck getting closer and closer, it freaks me out! You can't see it but you
can hear it. *lol* The ice cream truck is my paranormal phenomenon:
drawing in children to the wicked ways of sugar. It's all a state of mind.

My sister was the complete opposite of me. Candace had a Mrs.
Beasley doll. Eventually she left the doll behind and put on the glasses.
And didn't stop there. Candace became an excellent headhunter for the
financial district in both New York and Toronto. She and I agree to be
different. She believed I thought more like a girl because of my genetic
makeup. That I based my decisions more on intuition, she claimed,
showed I had more estrogen than she did. She thought more like a text
book and formed her decisions based on her intellect. Sisters growing
up in the same household – why do they turn out so differently?

There have got to be 25 possibilities to answer that question. Again,
it's all that state of mind. What if we could balance our intellect (what
we read) with our intuition (our gut feelings)? Why do we always have
to theorize to find the *shadow* – the bad part, the down side? Should we
be worried about inflation of the ego?

Why do we have to categorize or pigeonhole people? This person is
someone because they have a title? Does this person become a doctor
because he has a tested ability to read and write the exams with theory,
or do the doctors get their degree based on their ability to heal and
actually cure hundreds of cases?

We need the non-believers to entertain many new thoughts to bring
enlightenment to the forefront. Sure we need structure and boundaries
to protect people, but how much control is too much? We are all the
same; we all form part of this perfect Universe. We are all needed to
assemble the complete puzzle.

By listening to my inner self and striving to remain positive no matter what, I learned that the lessons, as hard as they were or hurtful at
times, were to improve my self-worth and knowledge to teach others. I knew I had to be as comfortable as possible. I learned to relax
and let go, to breathe. That there is nothing I needed to do but let the

sounds wash over me. I was going to be what I was going to be. My subconscious mind would work to change my life… it was in my blood from lives gone by. I learned to be pure in spirit. Inside was a place of confidence and security where all things are in perfect order with the Universe as I asked for it.

I don't have the Barbie and Ken life. I don't have time to sit around in my pajamas, and cry over spilt milk. The Universe pushed me harder and faster to wake up. I live far from what I witnessed as a little girl. I evolved and soon wasn't afraid of change.

The best advice is to relax and take slow deep breaths and go into yourself. Truth is apparent inside you, and far away from the clutter and clatter of the world.

The truth will guide you along your path. The Universal mind is perfect to rely upon for *all* of your affairs. Your every decision is answered from a perfect and abundant knowledge, through a law of attraction. Everything will come to you for your place at work, home and play. It's yours to draw upon.

Get this: everything that ever was and will be exists within you. All people, ideas and answers are in you. Divine intelligence is all around for you to call upon for your every need. There is no difficulty nor limitations. Create new experiences which you believe and accept, because the great reality is always good – and manifesting itself.

Do these concepts perhaps seem difficult for you to grasp and *believe?* Really, they are more logical than believing in a literal Garden of Eden with a magic apple and a talking snake, right? So many people believe in that Bible story to be an exact truth (it was supposed to be an parable – like a fable to teach a moral) because it was repeated to them so often and they talked about it. If you share your gradual awakening with others, that will help you connect and stay connected with these basic concepts of love, fear, energy, ego, spirit, intention, oneness with the Universe and so on.

The thoughts about your *things:* whatever is good, accept; whatever is not, ignore. For your concern is with truth and for understanding to expand. Your purpose in life is to reach outward and upward to abundance and unity.

Turn over each problem, one by one. You will have the confidence to evolve. Peace, love, balance, harmony, success and confidence are yours. Decide what you think and feel, for your entire life.

The avenues are always open to admit to the joy – it is waiting for you. Love all people; surrender your heart to humanity. The Universe will send you love and harmony back. Your reality is at the centre of your being for perfect love.

Refuse to accept anything but the truth. Just ask for it and it will happen.

You can achieve the power to receive the means and the way to get by, every day getting what you require. The Universe is infinite to your possibilities.

6 May 08, journal entry—

I want to be mainstream and normal all the time, to be accepted. Does this help? Sometimes it's hard being me with so much to say and do. Living in suburbia and going to the neighbors for tea and cookies can be challenging.

aka: Nadi, Dino

Birthday: July 20, 1965

Marital Atatus: Divorced

Last Place of Travel: Hawaii

Favorite song: *How Soon is Now* by the Smiths

Fav Artist: Tie between Prince and George Michaels (is that the healer in me?)

Fav TV show: *Grey's Anatomy*

Fav Saying: It's not over now, because they said the wrong thing. Or if they said the right thing – it's a good thing. (Martha Stewart is my hero. She's an angel!)

Fav Book: this one

Fav TV personality: Ellen

Fav Movie: *The Notebook*

MUSIC TRACK
Hear Journey singing 'Don't Stop Believin'
Just a small town girl
Livin' in a lonely world
She took the midnight train
Goin' anywhere

CHAPTER 14

Finger in the Socket

May 15 08, journal entry—
I am a conduit of energy. Information gets transferred to me and I am directed to deliver the message to the appropriate person for the highest and best interest.

Energy comes often when you least expect it. I find it amusing that spirit often travels through electronics. One day I wanted to shut off my energy work to sit and relax in front of the TV. A large pressure came over me and, from previous experiences, I knew this was a past life spirit. I stopped to listen: they were speaking Italian (which I don't).

The words and phrases repeat over and over in my head. They get louder. The pressure in my chest takes my breath away, to wake up and to stop watching TV to pay attention to the message. My physical body was led to call my girlfriend. I *had* to deliver messages in Italian to her. She was testing me and responded back in English. The spirit replied back in Italian.

My girlfriend started to cry and said there was no mistake that the spirit we were talking to was her father who passed away weeks ago. He had some unfinished business and messages for his loved ones. Passing on messages allowed him to move along his soul's journey.

When some people die, somehow their spirit gets stuck here on this physical plane, confused and possibly bitter or angry. Troublesome ones are called *adverse spirits*.

I have the ability to get rid of adverse spirits – that's what I was born to do – in homes, buildings, animals, plants and people. I purify and clear wherever I am and whatever comes my way. In order to do this I need to be pure light and love, have patience and kindness, and be very clear with the messages that come my way. If the message is strong enough, it will have the power to bring love and light through the power of intent. The mind is infinite to what it can see, feel, hear, touch and smell.

Recently I had a mansion for sale for an owner named David. This would be a ideal haunted house, priceless for TV. |NBC filmed there last week.| Spoons fly across the room. The doorbell rings and no one is there. This home is a stunning 6,000 sq. ft. Victorian Manor, decorated to the nines of the period. It's in the rural Ontario village of St. George.

How I was selected to sell David's home is an amazing journey in itself, and involves his previous house—

As a little girl I remember a recurring dream of an old home with winding stairs going up into the attic. Getting older I began to memorize the floor plan. After going down a wrong path in the dream, I discovered that I could get on the right path that led me up to the attic door that I was searching for. I realized I could *change* the dream which seemed *very* odd.

One night, now at the age of 35 years old, my dream became louder and more vivid. I could see the faces of the spirits in the attic, their clothes, I could hear the music, smell the scents, know the spirit had a message for me. I was not afraid for the first time. A spirit in the attic asked me to get out of David's house. Who is *David*, I wondered? I woke up and told my husband. It was an overwhelming feeling. I needed to tell someone for the first time that I had a recurring dream and it meant *something*. I wasn't sure what to do with this information but felt strongly I would know shortly what this dream meant.

The next day I went to work. An agent told me she was bringing, "an offer on David's house, one of your listings." My mind raced back to the details of the dream. Is this the David mentioned by the spirit? His home did have the same floor plan as in my dream. I was shocked that my recurring dream was playing out in the daytime. The home was vacant and I couldn't recall having a showing on this home yet, so where was this offer coming from? With tears in my eyes, I called my girlfriend Leanne and told her the story. I don't have time for this, I said, being a mom and high-paced real estate agent. I asked her if I was going crazy.

"No," Leanne replied. "You're just waking up like everyone else."

Leanne gave me a name and number of a friend to call who could help me with this phenomena. I chose not to and tried to go back to the world as I knew it. Yet I was intrigued and did want to know more – and so made a choice to explore the spirit world. My life hasn't been the same since this dream. There have always been signs. I just didn't see it before. It took the dream for me to fully realize I can be awake and aware of another force guiding us all. I paid attention closely from here on....

The agent brought an offer from a lady who claimed she was buying the home *because* of the spirit in the attic! The purchaser wanted to bring in a medium to explore what I thought at the time were *ghosts*. The similarities were unmistakable to what I saw in my dream. The spirit was now talking to me in this plane in the daytime – a calm voice inside my head. He had messages for me as to my past. This was getting interesting – I was thirsty for more.

When the deal closed, the house was officially sold, the new owners moved in... and the dream never came back.

After the sale of the home was finalized, I felt the need to tell David about the spirit and my learning. It was Valentine's Day when I visited David at his new house. He wasn't surprised by my comments since he had been aware of the spirit in the attic. That day a plaque arrived at his current home – it was from his passed loved one... a message for David. How it came to be delivered on Valentine's Day might be a mystery we never unravel.

David and I were grateful that we could relax and share the stories together. Were we brought together so people can live in haunted houses? Are there spirits in all the homes? All I knew was that David's life was colorful and full of experiences of laughter and joy. He was able to enlighten and bring so many people together through these magnetic homes. I was very okay with it too – after all, I now wasn't afraid of the spirit in that attic as I had been most of my life. I could now talk about it.

In David's current home (the Victorian manor), I have to catch my breath in several locations. My body wants to walk quickly past a room in the basement (it feels like a morgue). There is definitely energy that doesn't want me to be near the wine cellar. Upstairs, spirits live in the guest bedroom with a balcony. It's hard for me to go there too. Going upstairs into the attic is creepy. I find I cannot spend a lot of time in the bedroom in the attic next to the turret.

Every time I tried to send pictures of David's house to a potential buyer, my computer crashes. My doorbell rings, and when I answer no one is at the door. Lights flicker.

When David is at his home, the energy is calmer. I feel protected when David is in the same room as me. It might be a family member that wants David to stay in the home, I feel. They feel comfortable with him.

As I'm writing this, the angels are talking to me and want to explain! They are laughing out loud. *lol* They have a message from the manor spirits: the spirits say, once and for all they are tired of all the changes that have gone on in that building and want it to remain a home. David grounds the energy there, keeps things in balance. He is key. But I am sensing David is tired of that position and wants to move on. He's ready. The spirits are surrendering and want to let go, but are reluctant, they say. Misplaced events have happened there, they say. There is an original owner who has come back – something has to do with his spirit as well. Verbally abused his wife? Picking up on that energy. Something to do with a daughter carrying on the fortune and she didn't want too. Control issues at hand. Restless soul. There are many energies. Picking up on David's Grandma's energy too.

Picked these messages up from a distance – I haven't spent time in there to analyze the energy further. I'd like to get to the bottom of this as I would love to earn the large commission for selling this home!

I conducted an interesting clearing in Beverly Hills recently. The ultra-rich owners invited me in for a day to do healings on their family and friends. At one point, I stopped what I was doing and was drawn to a corner of the home. This house was once home to Fanny Brice (famed comedienne back in the 1920 and '30s). It was her energy, I sensed, that was interfering with the wife and was playing havoc with the furnace. I cleared the energy.

The wife related how a ghost whisperer tried to get rid of the energy before. That medium too felt it. She told Lauren to put *pods* in the windows of the home. I confessed to not knowing what *pods* were, but felt that candles and some incense might be calming.

Last Sunday was Mother's Day: every moment an event. In the morning my friend whispers to me, "You are like the mothership."

I didn't know what this meant. Was she referring to a Star Trek episode?

Three hours later, shopping downtown Toronto in Harry Rosen, my son Eric pulls out a T-shirt from the rack. He said, "Look, Mommy, this is for you. It says *Mothership* on the shirt."

I share a knowing glance with my friend. These signs happen so often when we are truly awake.

We go to lunch, sit down on a trendy patio, outside under the space heaters (Ontario doesn't know if it's winter, summer or spring). My children Eric Mercey and Jaxon Mercey, playing as kids do, are belly laughing to themselves. This one I couldn't read. I hear a lady behind us loudly say, "If it wasn't for all the *little mercies* out there, life wouldn't be interesting." *lol*

The boys settled and were surprised at her comment. I turn around – she appeared to be a lost soul, the homeless kind who had been swigging back the hooch. She was asked by the waiter to kindly leave when she tried to sell her diamonds for love at the table. Rather raunchy midday talk. My boys – the little Merceys out there – got an earful of social enlightenment.

My boys often remind me about the truths. Jaxon is a very perceptive boy… I've found that he is my benchmark in life.

He asked, "Why is it, Mommy, that the men in your life want to get to *us* to get to *you?*"

What was Jaxon saying? What did he see? He remembered when a man I dated bought him a Nintendo Wii and iPod Video Player, promised football tickets and a large big home where we could all live. Jaxon mentioned a recent offering of NHL playoff tickets.

Though only 13 years old, he could see they were trying to buy love. But he'd learned that their egos weren't going to get in the way of *his* life, not at his expense. He wasn't going to get hurt again. Jaxon had learned to live in the *now*. In this reality. Today we live in a modest 2,200 sq. ft. home. He is happy there, and wants to stay in that moment until he is ready to change it by his move away to college. Despite not having all the sports shoes he could want, Jaxon said we had enough money to travel the hard road, not the easy road. "There is a price to pay for the easy road. My Mom's heart."

There is nothing wrong with pruning people in your life. What he couldn't figure out was why were these men willing to try over and over, when they knew Mommy was… *different*. That was obvious to him and Eric.

This was a full circle moment-in-time for me to see how the strength and hard lessons of patience did pay off. My children respected their mother for choices made. My boys learned to respect others and to speak from the heart. They learned to be happy for what they grew to be… just to be.

At that very moment, I knew they would have all the values in them to choose the right mate for themselves when they were ready. I could release and surrender, to respect that Jaxon and Eric loved their Mommy and in turn they loved themselves to live in spirit. They would treat their women with kindness and comfort out of their own hearts, to fulfill their dreams with ease. They made me want to cry with pride this Mother's Day.

15 May, more journal entries—

Today I'm reminded of a key moment from years ago – after the awakening dream about the attic spirits (and my first situation of hearing spirit voices), I became increasingly more aware and sensitive to my surroundings.

My father came to see me one afternoon at my home.

He walked in. I could feel the pull. He wanted something. Something he didn't even know. My father just knew he could come to me to make himself feel better. He didn't care if I ended up feeling worse because of his presence or treatment of me. His ego enjoyed having power over me – control had been a lifelong pattern.

I clearly remember seeing his face change as I had asked him to leave my home almost immediately after coming into the kitchen. He said, "Have you lost your mind?"

I said, "No, I just found it."

A few days after that, the next person I had to stand up to was my husband. After a terrible marriage, the heartache went away as soon as I told my truth. Really I was having to stand up *to myself* – my past thoughts.

But this man wasn't willing to give up his fight so soon. I spent six years in divorce court after offering to help him. Years later I wanted still to help him. He refused. I learned an important lesson – you can't help those who don't want help. I walked away from him literally, moving with the boys to the next city. The boys have turned out so well.

By withdrawing (from my father, for example) and leaving (my ex) I believe I was a good role model to my sons. Ironically my absence helped these men become more aware of what was missing in themselves. It took a few years for my father to adjust to my new awareness. After that we communicated very well – there were new behavior patterns of communication between us. We learned to respect each other; his fears subsided as did mine. My father became a fine grandfather to my sons. He is truly a wonderful caring individual with more patience and kindness for himself and others now.

As I began writing this book and flowing truthful energy, my ex-husband began communicating and wanting to learn more. His fears subsided and he thanked me on my son's grade 8 graduation, offering congratulations on bringing up such a fine son.

∿

25 May 08, journal entry—

I'm not much of a TV watcher these days. However I was led to turn on the TV to a specific channel, 3/4 of the way through the final episode of *American Idol*. What I didn't anticipate was one of my favorite musical artists was appearing exactly at that moment in surround sound – Mr. George Michael. Was I just lucky to stop what I was doing and turn to the TV? No! It was bigger than that. I watched as Paula Abdul was standing, tears in her eyes. She, being as pure as I could read her, was as captured by his performance as I was.

The song he chose was perfect and fitting to what is happening in the world today and why I am writing this book. Paula got it. I got it. The message was clear. George Michael's thoughts or the vibration of his music gave me a rush of goosebumps, enough to stop me in my tracks!

How many people understand the importance to be aware of what is happening in our changing world? He sang the song *Praying for Time* from *Listen Without Prejudice*. Many millions have heard this song and those of other like-minded artists. Amanda Marshall, John Mayer, authors, artists alike – the message of peace and to clear the ego of what's polluting the world – we need to pay attention. This message can never be overstated or overplayed. Why do we need to be reminded? What are we doing to our society? What are we doing to ourselves? *Where Is The Love?* (– ask the Black Eyed Peas.)

The very next day I visit my friend TL. She is my esthetician who knows many of my stories (I will never live long enough to tell them all). After all the counseling and discussions, tears and heartfelt laughter, this young girl seemed bright and mature. She appeared to see the value in our talks! I asked TL, "Did you see George Michaels?"

She said, "Yes, my husband and I looked at each other and wondered when he would be finished, he had such weird glasses."

Sigh. She couldn't see what I could see. I had to respect her though; he didn't do it for her – everyone's awareness is awakened at different times through different messages and mediums. It's okay. There might be a country rock star, an author, a family member that's writing a message to their song now that will strike it with her....

She is young and has a new family, eager to get ahead in life and accumulate stuff. As I was thinking about raising the vibration of the planet, she was wondering what time Wal-Mart was closing. If she could walk a mile in my shoes – she'd see I'm trying to get *rid* of stuff. (Was I like this when I was her age? Did I really need to accumulate all those shoes? Yes, I think so.)

He is just a singer, entertainer, one of many, yet George Michaels did something special that night. To me a superstar is someone who can spread that message. Millions watch TV (especially that episode), so how brilliant to reach the masses to raise the vibration of so many? I certainly felt the peace. George, you are my hero! xo

Another enlightened soul in the media is Matthew McConaughey. He's just not another handsome face! Mathew was brilliant for moving the bedroom furniture of the 4 BR, 2-storey home to his living room. Then moving all the furniture out and selling his home to de-clutter. Then moving into a trailer in Malibu with his beloved surfboard. He could afford it all – did he choose to simplify to connect to his soul?

It's all around us; the media tells us so. We are all looking for that spiritual freedom. Whatever it takes to get there, is yours to discover. Downsize your home, upsize your lifestyle. What a concept!

---

25 May 08, more journal writing (emails)—

Hi Paula, it's been a while since we talked, but I wanted to thank you for all your encouragement and believing in me. Your insight and affirmation to my work, all those late night chats have paid off. It's been an amazing ride! Because of you and others I have met along the way, you all gave me the hope to see for myself. It was my own awakening as to who I really am. Remember the pains you were experiencing (and didn't know why)? Remember how they went away each time we connected? You gave me the strength to believe we can heal one another with the power of creative visualization and with, of course, the power of intent. With the right amount of intent to solve a problem, we can relax the body and heal our hearts and minds – the physical body just needs time to catch up.

It's been two years almost to the day when I saw in your eyes your past history. The blue eyes that came from an affair your great-great-grandma had with a Viking in the Azores. (I could see her, what she was wearing. I could tell you details of her life.) To give you affirmation of what you just came to realize yourself, remember that luncheon? I gave to you information you needed to hear, only to realize I knew nothing yet was teaching you everything you needed to hear. I realized that something else is guiding us to believe in spirit. I was helping to build your awareness and you in turn helped mine. We'd known each other for 15 years and had never shared these conversations before… Hhhmmm… why that moment? Timing is everything!

As a result of our efforts (sharing information, seeking truth), my phone hasn't stopped ringing – just as you said would happen. I'm receiving calls from people who seek the energy in the hopes to be well.

Today I receive a unique call. It was a call from Dr. Lorenzo Diana, a naturopathic physician – we have a client in common named Roy. Roy has a tumor on his liver. The tumor is so close to the only artery feeding his liver that it would be too dangerous to operate on to remove it.

Dr. Diana documents the blood flow, the energy shifts in the brain, Roy's energy levels. He was fascinated to find that instantly after Roy would have a session with me, Roy's physical body was changing.

Dr. Diana questioned me about my awareness of my abilities. These questions were similar to many asked before. How long have you known this? How long have you been healing people? How do you know these things? Why do you have this ability?

I think I have always been able to clear or purify energy. I just didn't know it. Over time, listening to people in my life, going within to find direction to keep me pure, listening to the children who speak the truth, watching the signs – all this helped me experience more and therefore believe more.

I can see through creative visualization methods to heal the physical body. I told Dr. Diana the following story about one of my early healings—

One day back when I was still a full-time real estate agent, I was asked to give an opinion of value on a home that was in my old stopping grounds of Brantford, Ontario. I hadn't sold real estate there in over six years. Why was I being called back there to help? There were other, local real estate agents who were more qualified than myself. I felt there were at least three other real estate agents in competition for the job. Yet if I spoke from the heart, I would be rewarded and get the listing.

This one was a little different. I was becoming more aware of my abilities to heal and intuitively knew this lady needed my help. I told my current boyfriend; he thought I was crazy.

The home was on a street where typically it was difficult to sell – six months might be needed to get the job done. This lady didn't know it yet but she was led to find me to help her with her physical pain. I knew also she wouldn't believe me and I needed to earn her respect in order to build her awareness.

Sure enough out of five agents, I got the listing and within days the home received an offer with perfect terms and conditions that suited everyone's needs. In fact this home was the highest-selling statistic on the street to date: sold in record-breaking time for $10,000 higher than the listed price.

The lady of the home was calling me constantly. She was legally blind and had been diagnosed with MS. She wasn't aware why, but she did know for some reason she was led to call when she was in pain. She told me I comforted her.

The secretaries back at the office thought I wasn't doing my real estate job very well because this seller was constantly calling, and with an upset voice. I knew I simply had to be patient and the seller would soon break down her barriers and realize what was happening here.

Always reading, I knew when a call wasn't really about the sale of the house, when she needed my healing help. Gradually I began to help her. I would send energy over the phone and ask how she was doing. She said better now, "I feel better when I talk to you."

I waited patiently for the opportunity to explain. Should I tell her? The time just wasn't right yet.

The next time you need me, I said, pick up the phone and please call me again.

The house sale conditions were waived and the house was sold, subject only to the buyers moving in. The seller called – she wanted me to help her get rid of her pain. The nurses couldn't come that day. I asked her if she wanted a visit from me and she said yes.

At her house I mentioned that it might seem a little unusual but I could try to send her energy to ease the pain. She liked the thought of this – she would try anything.

She laid on the couch and for five minutes I was sending her energy to the areas I felt needed repair. I directed the energy from a 20-foot distance. The vibrations were coming from my hands sending energy just above and along her limbs and torso. I could *see* the blockages. She instantly relaxed and felt the energy for the first time. She was aware this was working.

From the second floor a little boy about four years old comes down the stairs yelling. "Ah! Mommy, I feel tingling in my head. What's going on?"

This was getting interesting. Reading him while I was sending energy to her legs, I could sense he could see the energy. I asked the little boy what color am I. He replied *white,* without hesitation. I asked what color is your Mom, and he said *white.* When I asked what color is she normally, he said *pink.*

Mom's eyes were wide open in amazement at this demonstration of her son's abilities to see energy. He drew a picture for his mother of what he could see and feel. I left them to talk about it.

Reading her from a distance over a period of a week, I knew she was significantly better. One week had passed after the treatment with no verbal communication. Then she called and said she was playing basketball with her children. She was pain free and could also see the bank teller for the first time!

She didn't know how to explain this to her husband. He wouldn't believe, she said. I said that's okay – it was a gratuitous visit and I wanted to help you. She asked me what my fees would be if and when she could afford to continue the treatments.

"That seems like a lot of money," she remarked.

A month later, after the house had changed hands, I hadn't heard from her on the healing side of things. I did hear *about* her as the new owners were upset that the sellers' appliances didn't stay with the home. The seller I was representing took them. I made a nice, kind and clear call to the seller, explaining that it was written in the contract and they should remain. She had nothing else to say but agreed. I thought she and her husband would have been thrilled to get the price they did. I sincerely believed not only did I do an exceptional job for the seller, but I had reduced her pain as well.

The seller, however, called my broker-manager to complain that I took advantage of this situation as she was legally blind and I didn't read the contract to her. She wanted to pin me on this – I was the chosen fall guy. Her health restored (at least temporarily), this woman was again overly caught up in material possessions.

What was the lesson in this, I asked myself? This deal was pivotal for me. After that I chose to help people who needed and *wanted* the help, when they were ready and would *appreciate* it – and also to not spend my important time selling real estate.

I'd given up my ample real estate income, not an easy choice when I still had a monthly mortgage payment to make. I made the big step: taking out a line of credit on my home, devoting my time to concentrating on those who cared about healing and who would provide testimonials.

For the first time in my life I was stopping to see the flowers and bees all around me – things I couldn't see while being caught up in the materialistic world.

Dr. Lorenzo Diana's call led me to dig up the years of notes about my awakenings. I remember the energy being so strong that it forced me to immediately get a recording system to document Roy's and other healing sessions.

I had told Dr. Diana that anyone could transpire to build their awareness to heal. I had been able to take the time out to analyze it all and to practice. He could too. I could teach him through creative visualization exercises to help his clients. I wasn't special, I told him – just normal and *aware*.

He's anxious for our first in-person meeting. He's visualizing now the *magic* as he waves his hands across his clients' symptoms with ease, the disease disappearing. (I can sense his excitement and passion to heal with good intent.) I will share my information with him and any others who wish to heal with the highest and best interest.

MUSIC TRACK
The Clash playing 'Train In Vain'
Did you stand by me?
No, not at all.
This artist may have been blind and didn't see the signs. That's
okay. He's now found clarity (this is good) and is looking at self-
acceptance in a snap-shot picture. He's finally living in the Now.

CHAPTER 15

Balance and my kids

There are pages and pages of notes that I haven't looked at in years.
In fact I write and never really read what I write. Until now.

Back when I was still working from the real estate office, the book
peddlers who go door-to-door leaving books on speculation, hoping
someone will buy one, left a dream interpretation book. I bought it
for $10 and was now equipped and ready to receive the messages and
answers to the truth I was looking for. Only time would tell.

The dreams were intense. I wanted to pay attention to every little
detail to notice what I couldn't see for myself during the day. I couldn't
wait to go to sleep to dream and find the answers.

My son told me that you only get what you're ready to believe.

In the beginning I couldn't remember the dreams. I had to find a way
to wake myself up to remember and record them. So, before jumping
into bed, I would drink a half-glass of water and ask a question to be
answered in my dreams. I had the intent to be wakened to drink the
rest of the water and write with detail my findings on a piece of paper
next to my bed. This *worked!*

Eight years of recording dreams and other messages has proven them all to be accurate. Months before I would meet new people I would receive a full profile on these individuals and what the lessons were. It took me three years in the beginning to see during the day what I could have saved energy on if I only would trust my dreams. Wow, were they correct! I believed. I received more energy and more knowledge. I learned....

All this means, of course, is that we can also negatively influence the reality of our own situations with our conscious and unconscious thoughts. When we think negatively about our personal abilities, our looks or prospects in the future, these thoughts will influence how we feel and what happens to us in a very real way. We can make ourselves sick. Feeling off balance, without self-confidence, made me sick.

Jaxon, Eric and I are looking for a better way to balance our lives. We want to overcome the power struggle.

* * *

Now is the time in my life when I finally *get it*, when in the midst of all my fears and insanity, I've stopped dead in my tracks and am crying inside that *enough is enough!* Any guarantee of *happily ever after* begins with me. I am not perfect and not everyone will always love me, appreciate or approve of who and what I am. That's okay: they are entitled to their own opinions and views. I've learned the importance of loving and championing myself in the process and sense a new-found confidence of self-approval. I'm no longer complaining and blaming other people for things they did to me (or didn't do).

I've learned the only thing I can really count on is the unexpected. I've learned that people don't always say what they mean, and that not everyone will always be there for you, and that it's not always about me. I've learned that principles such as honesty and integrity are not outdated ideals of an era gone by – they are the mortar that holds together the foundation upon which you must build a life. I've learned that you don't have to know everything, that it's not my job to save the entire world and that you can't teach a pig to sing! I've learned to distinguish between guilt and responsibility, and the importance of setting boundaries and learning to say no. I've learned about love, how much to give, when to stop giving and when to walk away.

When times became grim, I knew I wasn't going down with a tin cup and never will.

Why do we feel that we have to be everything to everyone else? This pattern needs to change – was it learned behaviors? Isn't it amazing that we actually doubt ourselves... when we *know* we will have everything we possibly need?

＊

Everyone is a healer. When can we use those energies to heal ourselves?

Actually we do receive universal healing when we heal others. Yes, that's a good thing, but we must have integrity, have a conscience. Know your limits. Recognize the vibrations or discomforts and set your healthy limits and boundaries.

＊

4 June 08, journal entry—

Research on the Internet helped me put some pieces together quickly, to discover more in becoming aware on this life journey. I found that there were doctors recording healing phenomenon, people with illnesses were connecting and getting support from alternative sources, spiritual people are coming together to build strength to give others support in times of crisis. The demand is there, and teachers are learning more and more everyday what it takes to build programs to help those in need. These teachers of the spirit world are replacing their previous jobs with full-time healing positions. While there are fewer bookshelves in central Canada that provide this knowledge, my observation along the west coast tells me people there are ready and soaking it all up, wanting more. Why is this? If energy attracts the same.... When I went to California, people would walk up to me and say matter-of-factly that I was a healer. People who don't know you on the street, knew more than my family and friends did at that moment. Those are the people that make you a believer in yourself.

For example, a street vendor I met on Venice Beach befriended me. She left Toronto years ago to move to California. LA accepted her with open arms. It was acceptable for her to be herself and to connect with people off the street who needed her healing. They believed her there, more than her own family back in Canada.

On the radio in California, psychic network ads are playing constantly. People in the know may have many readers they call on (sometimes daily). These readers make good money advising clients what they can't see for themselves. The phone book has many pages of healers. They are everywhere. Is it the turtles, whales, the beach that draw these people to the coast?

There are some *excellent* healers in Ontario. I wonder why there isn't an excellent healing society to support them like there are in other parts of the world If these energy workers are born in these parts of Canada, should they stick it out and wait for the rest of their community to catch up in awareness? I would like to! (There is one sign of positive change: as I mentioned before, Therapeutic Touch is acceptable in some hospitals now in Ontario.)

I found a book (*The Children of Now* by Meg Blackburn Losey, Msc.D., Ph.D.) at a used book store up in Sauble Beach on Georgian Bay – there was an itsy bitsy shelf they classified as *New Age*. A book talked about *crystalline children, indigo children, star kids, angels on Earth,* and the *phenomenon of transitional children*. This doctor's research indicates an increasing number of children born with special energies. On the checklist of star kids, I found that I myself demonstrated all the enhanced psychic abilities: the ability to harness the subtle energy fields in and around the body, able to use earthly and cosmic forces to heal, gifted telepathic with others, can mentally see (clairvoyance/remote viewing), able to work outside time causing events to occur rapidly, sensitive to imminent earthquakes and other disasters, the checklist went on. One very interesting item I could relate to was that star children can often affect electronics or other electrical items, causing the items to malfunction. I am 43 years old, not a Child of the Now – does this research pertain to me? Could I look in the classified advertising section in my phone book and call someone to give me these answers? Why does it take years and years to find out who you really are? Can anyone be *defined*? Should we define ourselves – does it matter?

I've been asked these questions over and over and it seems that people need to justify reality by what they have read (their *intellect* tells them so). For me, I base my decisions on *intuition* – surely that's equally valid. As long as people are being healed and my work is for the highest and best interest, does it matter to define it all? Will I ever get through customs at the airport without questions? Will there ever be a category for someone like me? At least that would save me time and energy explaining to the people who check you with the electronic wands! After being interrogated through the many ranks at the airport, I needed to go through the electronic security scanner. All the belts, jewelry, metals were off the body. I still managed to beep, beep and BEEP every time. The lady officer asked, "Why do you beep so much – what do you do?"

I said I am a healer and explained the process of being detained at the intelligence agency. She stopped and wanted to hear stories of my healing. She started to cry and gave me a big hug and said, "God bless you. There should be more people like you in this world. Don't let them stop you. Keep going, honey!" (This was more affirmation it was okay to be me. Seems I didn't have to look it up in the phone book. It's the people on the street you get the answers from. Why do some people have to be so skeptical?)

Today's children are forming our new consciousness – if they have a voice to speak, we should listen. The innocence of children is bringing this into the mainstream. We should be grateful for all the children in their loving grace who have come to help us transition in this new world. Their mission in life is greater than us all.

I have seen many children awaken (re-awaken!) to their levels of consciousness. Children need help to understand they aren't alone in their beliefs. Believing their senses, their thoughts, feelings, visions – the children do not need to fear. They need to know that they are loved and everything about their existence is perfect. That they are a part of this grand plan in the Universe to purify. We are a part of *their* puzzle, for us to learn. If they respect themselves, there is less fear. Thus their vibrations are free to rise to raise the rest of the world's vibrations to a better place. Sickness and disease ceases, and they grow up healthy.

My younger son was tested for autism, hearing and learning disorders by specialists. Jaxon couldn't focus on his environment – he focused on what he wanted to do without fear. I could not allow Jaxon to get out of my sight. As much as I and his caregivers would understand his behavior, Jaxon managed to escape from us all. At the tender age of one and a half, Jaxon would unlock windows and the screens of our home (as we kept the doors locked) and Jaxon would be found running in his diaper with no shoes down the street... laughing out loud. I remember the time when he disappeared from the fenced-in pool area of the Brantford Golf and Country Club. Jaxon was found streaking down the second fairway... a golfer brought him back to the pool.

At the age of 2-1/2, Jaxon managed to escape from his ski school teacher, somehow wandering off to the chairlift on his own. Jaxon convinced the chair attendants to stop the lift and pick him up to put him on the chair. I had to use my intuition to see if he was alright – I believed he was. We saw Jaxon coming down, snowplow style with a *big* grin on his chapped face. Whoa, Jaxon just came down a black diamond hill! Oh my! (His older brother had tears flowing down his face, crying in fear for his brother. *He's doing it again, Mommy. Stop him!*)

The doctors wanted to put Jaxon on ADHD medication. They told me that if I didn't, by the age of 17 Jaxon would be in jail. I declined and instinctively knew there was a better way to harness his energy without the drugs. If Jaxon needed to take this medication for a long period of time, I didn't trust the medicine. What implications and side effects would there be by the time he was 17? I needed to be more aware and find a better solution for Jaxon to overcome his behaviors.

When Jaxon was five, I began balancing and centering his energy. Jaxon's behavior calmed. He was happier and more content. Jaxon began co-operating and paying attention in school.

I worked with Jaxon on my own in his early years. Without medication and visits to the doctors, Jaxon is now a very capable, loving, handsome, 6-foot blond, blue-eyed, 14-year-old. He resembles actor Leonardo DiCaprio. MVP football star playing with kids three years his senior, 90 per cent average. Jaxon models, sitting patiently for directors all day while shooting commercials. He loves to travel, socialize and has many wonderful friendships. Thank god I didn't let him be drugged with ADHD medication! Jaxon broke his finger recently while playing volleyball at school. The surgeons spoke about operating and putting a pin in. My intuition kicked in. I gave the surgeon a disappointed look and asked how much time do I have to heal the finger before they had to operate? They gave me two weeks. Within that two-week period I sent energy to Jaxon's finger, and he drank antioxidant, anti-inflammatory juices filled with nutrients such as the acai berry, glycuamine and other ingredients to rejuvenate new cell growth. This mix of juice from the Brazilian rainforest makes no claims that it is a cure or prevents any disease. It is not a drug but a blend of fruit juices that are good for you.

Did the collagen-building properties help Jaxon to heal his finger? Or was it Mommy's healing abilities? Yes, done in two weeks. The x-rays showed significant improvement. Jaxon escaped surgery and being down for the summer with a pin in his finger taking months to heal. If he'd had surgery, there was a possibility that his finger would stop growing as well.

A few years ago I realized I myself showed some of the classic symptoms of mild autism. I found myself talking to someone and then realized I was channeling messages. Information was being downloaded to me in multiple states of mind at once. I would repeat words, or get stuck. My boys found a way to pull me out of my dazed state of mind. I couldn't recall the conversation I was initially having but could recall my children counting 8... 9... 10! But what I did remember was some specific detail: a picture image or information that was being given to me to repeat at the right moment. Over time I learned to control and to train the energy that was coming at me from different sources.

I've always been sensitive to my environment. My first automatic angel writings said to wait for the world to catch up before publishing these items. I respected the energy and did. With one week left to go to writing this book, both my computers crashed! Being a clairvoyant and writing visions with ease for eight years, I still managed to question myself. Should I actually publish this information? Was the electro-magnetic energy interfering with this process – should I stop writing? Out of fear I started second guessing my journey (as we humans so like to do). How am I going to pay for these new computers? Future Shop has a 12-month, no-payment plan… *lol* More credit? Jeesh….

What will others think of this book? Am I actually shifting and becoming overly concerned with what others will think of me? I needed to get back to *me*!

Nevertheless, I called a friend to seek her approval. She boosted my vision that led me to conclude that *success* is merely another word for *balance*.

Everything has to be equal. You do what you're meant to do. In your heart and in your mind. We have a problem in our society: we tend to make decisions out of fear (or jealousy, a cover-up for fear in ourselves). We should instead stop that and be the best we can be, and stop beating ourselves up with jealousy, self-doubt and worry. Smile, be happy and that's that. Sure this book will have criticism. But, I laugh to myself: the person with no money or fame has little pressure and nowhere near the balance to maintain compared to those in so-called higher places with huge material fortunes.

A lot of people would like to be Donald Trump or the President. The question is would they like the balancing part of the equation? Most only crave one side of it – the power, fame and riches. However life is a mathematical equation, with two sides. Most perceive only the appearance of success, not the downsides.

My mind just downloaded the angel writing I received years ago on the 10th Commandment – about not coveting others' possessions, family and situation. Could the Bible just be common sense, the teachings of Jesus being information that was downloaded to him, to help us awaken to Universal truths about oneness and love?

That concept speaks of the *lack of balance*, of the self-perpetuating situations, the roller coasters we put ourselves on.

Does happy require medications?

How do we get help riding up that hill?

Can we go down twice as fast?

Be careful of what? Does it matter? Why can't we just be happy with ourselves – for this moment is perfect in time?

Should we then live like it's the last f—kn' day of your life? *lol*

It's all about balance. And love.

Listen to Mariah Carey, Beyoncé, Mary J. Blige, Rihanna, Fergie, Sheryl Crow, Melissa Etheridge, Natasha Bedingfield, Miley Cyrus, Leona Lewis, Carrie Underwood, Keyshia Cole, Leann Rimes, Ashanti and Ciara in 'Just Stand Up – To Cancer'

Everything will be alright, yeah
Light up the dark, if you follow your heart
An inspiring song for those battling disease.

CHAPTER 16

Healing notes

June 4 08, journal entry—

I have been receiving positive feedback and have had doctors who want to learn more about this energy working process. Roy is the client I mentioned before who has been battling cancer and has a tumor next to the only artery feeding his liver (he had a 70% liver resection in 2003). He visits once a week for an hour session at a time. Within the first treatment Roy noticed improvement in his physical appearance and had more energy to get through his day. His doctor reported instant changes:

Hi Nadine,

Roy has been a patient of mine for the past 4 years. We have been using nutritional supplements and detoxification for Roy's treatment. We have been using electrodermal screening to monitor his progress. What I have noticed with the particular treatments you have been giving is that there are physiological changes in his liver and blood flow following his treatments. I will keep monitoring his progress.

Dr Lorenzo Diana, Naturopathic Doctor

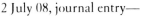

2 July 08, journal entry—
Sorry for not writing in this journal for a while. Kids' graduation, end of school year, and got bombarded with energy I was trying to balance.

I've had a setback (one could easily end up in the hospital with the symptoms I had in the last four days). I suffered from what some would call fatigue, migraine headaches to the point of shutting all light out, cold cloths on my head, fever, pulse vibrations in my head. Couldn't breathe or sleep for 4 days. The pain was excruciating!

There are adverse energies that once or twice a year I battle, yet learn from. I can remember these symptoms since I was a little girl of five years old. As I battle these forces, I get downloaded more energy, more vibrations and then the ugly symptoms subside.

By the fourth day, I usually end up vomiting, sweating, burping out the adverse energies and getting replenished with cooling, tingling, calming energies. The next day I am back being myself, fully charged to do a 2-hour vigorous workout and ready to heal again!

It's a tiring process but it's well worth the gain in the end....

Something out there doesn't want me to have these energies to heal, I feel. They certainly try to shut me down and strip me of the power at times.

30 July 08, journal notes—
I met Henry in Hawaii in March and had a 45-minute session with him. I scanned his body and could detect something he needed to check with his medical doctors. He hadn't had any symptoms so ignored my advice and didn't have any medical diagnostic of this location in his body.

Yesterday I worked on Henry from a distance (he lives in Vancouver and I am in Ontario). Every healing session has a beginning and an end. At the start it is important to ground and protect the energy between the client and myself. Some instantly feel the power of intent to center the body as if they have gone to yoga. And in the end they should breathe easier, be more relaxed and expect their skin to feel cooler. Intuitively Henry knew I would make his tummy rumble and get things moving. (I didn't know why. I just knew that's where the energy would go. That's where he needed it.)

It's all vibrational energy. My energy velocity goes up to receive high vibrations to send out to the client. I can get very clear and distinct messages at this point to help guide the individual. I do need to respect their level of awareness but some clients do wonder and their thoughts go through my mind as I am guided. Through the power of intent, some clients will feel, see or hear a *presence* responding directly to these questions or thoughts about how to improve their soul's health. That presence would be their own guide or angel.

In a healing, when the chakras have been opened and the body is aligned, I am guided to check the soul – do they have all their energies with them? Are there energies that are interfering with their true soul, life force energy? Are they clear and pure to the best of their abilities? Can we bring more energy to give them clarity and focus? Should we remove the adverse blockages to promote clarity?

I tend to hear and am guided as to what is happening on a soul level. Once we bring the soul to its highest potential, the mind, body and soul tend to release and surrender the blockages, and the body is ready to receive more energies to manifest and open up opportunities. Are they balanced? Are the centers to be perfectly aligned? Do we need to send energy to the meridians? I'll have visuals of sending energy and can *see* the chakras opening up. I had to go read some books to help explain what I see and what naturally just happens, to communicate on some standard level for others to learn or understand. The energy I can bring is always specific for what that person requires at that moment. Their soul speaks and the energy comes through myself as a natural and pure conduit. I deliver the energy to them. I don't usually have to consciously think – it's mostly better if I don't. There is no form of control on my part. I don't usually get tired because it's not my energy – the energy is here for whomever wants to receive it for themselves. Some who understand this call me a 'soul doctor'. When you change your soul vibration you can start to heal yourself.

For Henry his soul was fine (I got a *check, check, check*).

Usually the energy travels to the base of the spine and into (what I understand) is the nervous system. Up the spine to a sensory spot at the base of the skull where the neck joins. Travels down the arms. Then I am guided to send energy at the ankles up to the hips. That way the energy, the voices tell me, gets more quickly into the immune system, hence the blood stream to the cell level.

As I was guided and protected, the energy for Henry missed the usual check points and was flowing not just with one hand but two hands this time directly to the stomach area. During a distance energy healing session, my hands are moving over a visual of the client's body in my mind. Somehow the energy is moving to the person as if we were in the same room, not 3,000 miles apart. I asked Henry if his stomach was upset; he said no. I trusted my intuition as my hands don't allow me to move them (I respect the energy and direction that my physical body is aiding another). I was guided to send large amounts of energy to a specific area near the stomach. He could sense things moving around in the abdomen.

I didn't know why at this time that it was so important to send energy to Henry's abdomen when usually I start off sending energy to the spine.

Coincidently(?) I received three emails the very next morning with information on how the immune system is helped by probiotics and prebiotics. I combined the info – getting confirmation inside about its validity – and sent this message to Henry as advice about building a healthier body:

Did you know that it is estimated that 60% of your immune system is located in your gut? The healthier I eat, the less frequently I get sick, and the less frequently I get digestion problems.

The aim is to build up both prebiotics and probiotics – not from supplements but from regular natural foods.

Probiotics are basically live microorganisms (friendly bacteria and other good microorganisms) in certain fermented and raw foods that can be ingested. Some probiotics you may have heard of are bifidus, lactobacilli, L. casei, and so on. It's estimated that the average person has several *trillion* of these little helpers working at any given time inside his or her digestive system.

Probiotic microorganisms actually thrive in the acidic environment of your stomach and small intestine, and provide tremendous benefit to you: improved digestion; increased immunity; help in reducing yeast infections, urinary tract infections, etc.; reduced chances of diarrhea and/or constipation; improved lactose tolerance; increased absorption of vitamins, minerals and other nutrients; and increased production of white blood cells to help reduce inflammation, allergies and other conditions.

Keep in mind that taking antibiotics kills off a portion of the friendly bacteria living inside of you, so you need to make sure to increase your intake of probiotics if you ever feel compelled to take antibiotics. Many medical doctors will carelessly prescribe antibiotics even if you have a viral infection (which is pointless). This is only doing you harm by killing some of the good probiotic bacteria in your system and potentially allowing another bug to make you ill now that your defenses are reduced.

Foods that are good sources of health-giving friendly probiotics include these:

- plain yogurt
- kefir (similar to yogurt, but more of a liquid form of fermented milk)
- aged cheese – blue cheese, hard aged cheeses, aged cheddar
- kambucha – a type of fermented tea (this has a very strong taste, so consider mixing it with regular iced tea)
- natto, miso and tempeh – forms of fermented soybean
- sauerkraut – probably needs to be homemade as most supermarket sauerkrauts are pasteurized, which kills the friendly probiotics.

While probiotics are the actual organisms, *prebiotics* are types of foods that you can eat to help stimulate the growth of probiotics within your system. Traditional dietary sources of prebiotics include soybeans, inulin sources (such as Jerusalem artichoke, jicama and chicory root), raw oats, unrefined wheat, unrefined barley and yacon.

This morning Roy was in for his weekly session. He went yesterday to Buffalo, New York for a newer product (Erbitux, not yet approved in Ontario) that apparently has a 20% success rate in fighting cancer. Roy started this treatment a month ago. The session was very different today after his drug treatment. I found his body to be very toxic, so I was releasing a lot (many, many burps). I had the sense that his body was saying *enough already!* Today I could clearly see a visual of the enzymes as if they were being shattered and dispersing inside the stomach areas. Then another visual came and it was as if cylinder-like tubes were being formed together after a cleansing scenario. I was getting a message as if these cylinders were the molecules pairing in the enzyme. The enzymes were forming stronger bonds in the body to disperse the cancer cells. I had no knowledge of this information before and asked Roy if he could explain what I saw.

He said to his understanding that this is the process to fight off or kill the cancer. The cancer doctors check and monitor the blood for the level of a glycoprotein molecule called CEA (carcinoembryonic antigen). That level was up when he first realized he had a tumor. The MRI confirmed the tumor. Now the CEA levels are coming down, indicating those enzymes are dying off in the blood stream. The enzymes making up the tumor are bursting through the explosion of this light energy and the debris is moving out of the system. Meanwhile good enzymes are joining together to strengthen the liver. When you take something out, you replace it with good. I could *see* the energy explosion getting rid of the old enzymes.

Roy went from over 20 CEA level in December; he is now down to a 3. The peripheral issues were dealt with in our first sessions, then within two weeks the enzymes levels dropped drastically. Who knows for sure, but Roy believes the biggest factor of the decrease in CEA levels, indicating the tumor is becoming inactive and being killed off, is not the medical treatments but our energy sessions. Roy feels that the drug Erbitux may have stabilized the tumor growth but it's the energy work that reduced the tumor and cancer cell count. Roy's belief is that the count will be down to a zero in the next few days.

Talking about this with Roy on the phone just now, there was a squeal and loud screech, then Roy's phone just died! Weird. He called me back on his cell. Weird. That my phone was not to be available for him to call me back was weird too. (Another healer was calling in from Vancouver at that very moment. Hhhhmmm.)

Mischa had been diagnosed with 4th stage pancreatic cancer on October 1st, with cell counts of 375 and a large tumor. Within four energy healing sessions and combination Chinese greens and off and on sessions with chemo, Mischa has proven to be one of the rarest cases today. The doctors call Mischa's recovery a miracle. His cell count is a *zero.*

While waiting for a healing session, Mischa experienced my coffee maker surging with energy, and turning on spontaneously. Lots of energy in that room!

The next day a large former NHL hockey player, Peter Zezel, came for energy healing. Perhaps I needed more energy because of his size. That may account for why my home's alarm system surged with energy, blew and needed repair.

Doesn't Donna call me that night with a message from up above:
Your job is to manage the energy that comes down. Blowing circuits is a waste of power. [No kidding. Not to mention extremely expensively frustrating.]
The higher level of concentration is faster and more intense and awakening of the body at that time. Extra energy is filtering off. You need to learn to control it better. Hold your hand up to the sky and release it. No manuals are written for you, Ms Mercey. You can't open up the book and turn to page 5 on how-to. Energy goes within a few days. If any extra, sending it back up. The radio waves are interfering with conditions on Earth. Get rid of the energy residual. Or look out to the street and send it to the unhappy neighbor. lol
Lights go off in front of you. Sign to release the energy. People who are in the know think it's hot to blow lights. A true sign that they are operating

on high level is that energy should be in control. Keep palms up to the sky as
you have been guided and send the residue back.

On my birthday I wanted to treat my family to the movies. Angelina
in *Wanted* was playing. It's time to curve some bullets! I go up to elec-
tronically pay and get there with fingers crossed when the machine
goes down and freezes. Not only did mine but the whole bank of machines froze.

My Dad now gets it and says, "You stay away from machines."

He paid with cash, which I guess is okay, since it was my birthday,
right?

I can get specific detail and see right down to a cell and molecule level and get messages for affirmation either for the client or myself if
needed.

The testimonials speak for themselves but what if we could teach
this to others to help them creatively visualize for themselves? Or help
doctors to understand how the mind, body and soul are connected?

To help a sore arm could have everything to do with the mind and
how the body stored adverse energy from the shock or trauma associated with an accident. To heal requires more than surgery and pills.
A lady called me from a town 2.5 hours drive away – she had heard
about me and wanted to believe but didn't understand the process. I
sent her energy from a distance over the phone as we chatted. She instantly felt different and knew to trust to believe. (We only get what
we are ready to believe.) For almost three years she had suffered from
a painful shoulder/arm ailment. She tried everything. Surgery, doctor
after doctor, acupuncture, massage therapists… nothing worked. She
was tired of not being able to wash her own hair, drive a car or even
the simple task of raising a fork to eat. Intuitively I knew I could help
her, and release the energy stuck in one of her states of mind, without
touching her. Scanning the body with my mind and energy I released
that blockage. Her arm rose up without pain for the first time in years.
Her goal was to be able to go on vacation. She went.

There have been many others with chronic pain where they can't work or function normally so their family life is interrupted. Through word of mouth I have been able to touch hundreds and make a difference to change their lives.

In Roy's case of having cancer on his liver, I knew I had to send energy to all the sensory organs and look after the whole because one organ's function relies on the other. Channeled information today is coming through: *You can't just radiate that area, you* need *to look after the blood flow throughout the body to purely release the toxins in that area. Stabilization is required in that area for sure but the body, mind and soul need to regroup on a whole to beat the cancer. It all starts in the mind and the soul. It's the physical body that catches up to us over time to talk to us to say, Hey! Wake up!*

How do I know this? I know I am not the only one. There have to be many, many more out there who are born with higher frequencies for a very good reason. Some are unaware of their abilities or hiding from the reality.

I keep putting an intention out there to manifest so I'll be able to find these people and bring awareness to them. The message is they should not be fearful with their knowledge and that we need to believe in so much more!

They are coming. I don't know how I am finding them but healers are out there! Here's my story of meeting someone on the street just like me...

I was led to a store called *Goodness Me*, a natural organic store. I didn't have enough money at the time to buy anything but I was led to examine products I hadn't noticed before and was captivated by these brown cardboard boxes sitting on a shelf labeled Jordan Detox. There was nothing flashy or pretty about the packaging. I was definitely led to learn more about the content and benefits of this product that possessed high potential to help clear disease. Connecting the dots I remember a visual of me supplying Dead Sea Salt and other products to clients after a healing session; the packaging showed it was prepared in Hamilton, Ontario (my home base). Also sitting in the healing room I would channel and get messages that for clients and especially cancer clients, a detox product would aid them after a healing session and work to their benefit. They *needed* to get rid of toxins in their body. Not only did they need to balance their body with nutrition, raise their PH levels, reduce acid properties in their body, but the body needs specifically to get rid of the toxins.

Wondering where this angel nudge would lead me, I decided to do some research in other stores. That evening I went to a health products store and instantly felt a presence, a wonderful calming. The girl explained the owner wasn't here, so I knew I had to come back tomorrow.

Initially planning on hitting the store at 10 a.m. when it opened, I found myself wanting to delay going, for no particular reason. Instead I worked out on my air climber.

Just after 11:30 a.m. I arrived and introduced myself to another customer. Here was a lady who looked *just like me* (same curly blonde hair, brown eyes, her mannerisms, the way she tilted her head to hear). I needed to ask her what she did for a living – not wanting to be too forward, yet I felt her gravitation towards me as well. Sharon is her name. Sharon turns out to be living a parallel life to mine: divorced, children of the same age, relationships gone wrong. Sharon had very calming energy. She opened to me and I knew she was reading me as I was reading her. Openly as if there was no one in the store and as if we had known each other for years, we were communicating messages for one another. Wow! Talk about electricity. I could feel the presence – it was something to pay attention to and to trust. I knew I had to help bring out her awareness.

The storekeeper Janice opened up the dialogue further and said Sharon is a nurse and wonderful registered message therapist. I read Sharon and said, "You see the internal body as I see it."

She said yes.

"You have negative and positive charge hands independent of each other and you read people like I do to help them."

She said, "Yes, how did you know?"

Sharon was shocked as she usually doesn't talk about this side of her. I thought if she was more confident about her abilities to network with other healers on this level, she would have so much more to offer and give. Sharon had great talent! We exchanged cell phone numbers. Wow, I thought, a new friend to learn from and to exchange thoughts.

Sharon read my body, seeing a cist and then asked, "Why do you work on everyone else but forget to heal yourself?"

This was amazing because I was scheduled to have an ultrasound the following Monday to check on a cyst in my abdomen. I didn't have any symptoms but my medical doctor, knowing my psychic abilities (and quite skeptical about all this), wanted to see if the cist I had previously was any larger.

I went for the ultrasound and the cyst was still there. Sharon said I could heal on my own but I need to concentrate more. She wanted to help. The doctor will probably want to get rid of it her way: drugs, surgery… Decisions to make. Between Merlot and a Cab?

I have the true diehard clients who know more about the cosmic forces than I do. I guess I am still learning about Saturn in Uranus. They will call to book appointments close to the full moon and know that my energy is at its highest then (go figure, *lol*) to be enlightened with the divine forces that be. Most have never experienced such high energy before. I get many invites to come to group meditations. I usually decline and I am not sure why….

MUSIC TRACK
Stevie Wonder performing 'Superstition'
Very superstitious,
Nothin' more to say
Of course for those sitting on the fence: how can you believe in
things you don't understand? Just breathe, release and accept.

CHAPTER 17

Dirty Harry thinks I'm a keeper

July 30 08, journal entry—
My friend Mike is here from Vancouver to visit and then he'll go to Detroit to hang out on the set of a movie Clint Eastwood is filming. They have been long-time friends.

Mike has lived a colorful life and is a lot like me in that he meets the best of the best and networks to bring people together. I'm grateful to Mike for the doors he has opened.

Mike's stories are so unique that they are sometimes hard to believe. Mike tells an LA fitness trainer for the stars about me. It is a small world: the trainer tells Clint that I am a phony baloney clairvoyant who doesn't know anything. Word trickles back to me. I've never met the trainer, but I've talked to Clint on the phone. Why do I sense some explaining needs to happen? Do I need to? Am I suppose to? Will I have to live like this for the rest of my life? I do know there is something universal happening out there. And, yes, even in sleepy Ontario, people are searching for more. For answers to the hidden truths. To the secrets that guide us.

Then I think: it's okay. That's all he may know. You only get what you're ready to experience. You only experience what you are ready to see and believe. We are made up of different fabrics. Different beliefs. It's all good.

Will I actually be given that opportunity to meet Clint in person this week? If so, could Clint be the one to help awaken the masses?

30 July 08, second journal entry—

Couldn't help notice the time I sent the last email – 1:11.

The stenographer who is helping me transcribe the recordings of some healing sessions (I intuitively picked her out of the phone book) believes in psychic energy, and has asked for answers to come into her life. So we are trading services.

2 August 08, journal entry—

No Clint...

Mike said he was staying on the movie set with friends. All his friends, Mike said, they are having so much fun, that he can't get them off the set.

So no invite for me to meet Clint in person after all. Hhhhmmm. Something's just cool with me. It's all the little stories and affirmations. More dots to connect for my awareness. Is it meant to be that I actually meet Clint?

Last night Sharon came over to go out together for dinner. We both agreed it was very difficult in the beginning to look at each other's eyes and have a discussion without looking away. Sharon equally was in awe about the similarities and the instant comfort we felt – as if we had known each other for years and years.

We talked and talked, and usually interrupted each other as messages would flow freely – kind of spooky for both of us. Sharon wanted to grab her cigarette which she admitted was an unhealthy choice of a crutch; I wanted to swig another sip of red wine.

The energy was flowing between us; I was burping (which she thought was cute) until the barriers and fears subsided.

For a change I didn't want to go out for dinner! It was much more relaxing to me to whip up a lovely meal here and stay in my element of comfort.

Sharon watched me prepare the meal and noticed my aura changed significantly. Colors were morphing! As she asked questions the energy around my head would change. When I answered her about some past issues, the energy would be darker. When I spoke about my new business adventures, my head would light up! Sharon's explanations confirmed that I needed affirmation about my own self-worth and direction.

After a pesto-brown rice-veggie pasta, Sharon tried to teach me to see the color between fingers by concentrating. I still couldn't. I told her my talents require me not to see. Somehow I knew I wouldn't be able to do what I do without fear if I did see color. The feeling and hearing aspect while my eyes were open was good enough for me.

I asked Sharon to sit in the chair where clients sit and also where I watch TV in my down time. She said, "You don't know what down time is. Your mind is always going like mine. When you go to a show you probably see the energy and thought vibrations coming out of people."

I said, "Yes, I feel that energy and hear it."

Sharon sat in the brown chair and watched the pilots I did for a TV show and documentary. The film piece was meant to shock and intrigue viewers about paranormal energy.

She was polite and continued to sit there until the paranormal pilot DVD was over. I offered to send energy and she said, "No, maybe another day. This night is more than I can handle and I need to process all this."

Sharon's eyes changed and looked spooked as she said *the chair is vibrating*. I told her it doesn't vibrate. So I sat in the chair and had *never* felt it like that before. The chair was filling with energy without me trying.

When she knew this didn't feel normal for me either, Sharon felt some comfort and we waited for the energy in the chair and room to settle. She was glad she did experience my energy working and said she had never experienced such a force before in her five years of work, not even in a large group mediation.

She was now at ease and didn't question the chair vibration. She just knew that great energy was in the room. She commented that my Grandmother who had passed would come to clear the energy residuals from the room to help me if I didn't. I knew this to be true – more affirmation.

We discussed dreams, how our messages come to us, how we translate them to those who need them. We read for each other and gave insight into each other's lives, in an equal manner. She said that the tummy issues (the cyst) were to awaken myself to *honor thyself* and let go of the past. That I could heal myself. This I knew but I am still human with fears and needed to be reminded and certainly needed that affirmation from up above.

Sharon has difficulty in her nursing job because of conflicted interests and viewpoints. She's a natural healer and sees some of the barbaric medical healing methods further toxifying our systems.

We had so much in common: looks, personality, interests. We were grateful to have met each other. She came as a new friend and we both left more enlightened than before. I wonder just how will she describe this experience to her friends?

My girlfriend Norma invited me to a hockey charity event at the local Yuk Yuk's comedy club. I *knew* I had to go to make a connection to help someone.

I was enjoying the conversation and rapport of the gentleman and his wife sitting next to me – Keith and Karyn. Keith asked me what I did for a living. Pausing as always, I went within and asked if and how much to say (depending on the person's level of awareness). I was giving a go-ahead, that it was quite necessary to speak my truth.

Next Keith takes my card and says, "I will be calling you to help a dear friend in the hospital."

I went within, then answered his question very confidently that, yes,

I could make a difference and would help. I mentioned to Keith that usually I get picked on and hope the comedian doesn't ask what I do for a living.

Doesn't the lead comedian pick on me! Centered me out and asked me what I do for a living. *lol* I told him I was a real estate agent – yes, the easy way out! I was now on the stage and the center of attention in front of hundreds of people not just once but between each act. I allowed my intuition to kick in and began reading the comedian host and played him before his every gesture. We managed to put on quite a show for the crowd.

He asked me if I had ever done this before. I said no, of course not.

People were coming up after and thanking the comedians for making them laugh so hard and wanting to meet me. *lol* Other real estate agents were coming up to me, giving me their cards hoping to network. *Ugh,* not as much fun.

About one week later I received a call from Lisa (Keith's friend who needed help for her husband Pat) to visit the long term care hospital in Burlington. I sensed I could help further and needed to go. This was my first hospital client visit.

Lisa closed the curtains in the room and I was free to close my eyes, move my hands, breathe and certainly burp without interruptions.

I was reading that Pat was hungry. Energy was flowing in large forces directly to the brain and spine areas of the body. I could *see* just as well in this hospital setting as when I have been working with people in my home. Lisa was pleased as I answered her questions about advice she was getting from other people and the doctors.

I told her Pat only needed to see me once a week and we could make a difference in three months.

Pat had suffered a heart attack and a stroke to the brain. At one point, Pat had *flatlined* on the monitoring machines – essentially dying – then chose to give life another chance. I acknowledged that his physical organs were fine and could see the difficulties in the brain and spine. Pat had been hooked up to a feeding tube as his refluxes wouldn't allow him to eat or drink.

My session was on Thursday for one hour in the hospital.

Lisa called two days later with excellent news. Pat drank most of a whole bottle of water without gagging – the first time in a year – and looked at her with such conviction and belief that he was obviously improving! Paul was smiling to Lisa. His eyes were talking to her. Tears of joy filled Lisa's eyes.

I was hired to continue to send energy to Pat to help his mind and body. I told Lisa his spirit was just perfect! I could speak to Pat and transcribe his thoughts to Lisa. This man had the will and life-force to get better!

- ❧

3 August 08, journal entry—

Mike was at a BBQ in Detroit with friends and was outnumbered by the divorced women who he claimed were men-haters. They decided to pick on Mike who is 52 years old and never been married. He was telling his male pal that his girlfriend (me) would never talk like that and is perfect and calm and patient all the time – *no matter how irritating I can be*, he said.

As a result I received an invite to go down to the next BBQ on Sunday and meet his friends (possibly for back up against those women?). Healer to the rescue!

Mike said we could stay over and go to the set to meet Mr. Eastwood himself. Hhhmmm… just as I was hoping for an *out* to this relationship, and had my mind made up. The downside is I am a healer trying to be positive and make it work. Will I actually meet Clint this time as Mike promises?

- ❧

8 August 08, journal entry—

Finally had a great meeting with Clint, hours before my flight to Vancouver for an Alaska cruise. Here's how it unfolded—

One hour into the drive towards Windsor I'm thinking of Mike, our relationship, and being late for the BBQ. I forget that I'll be crossing the border to the Detroit movie set and might need a passport. I turn around....

Back in the car speeding towards the border a song is in my head. Daydreaming of the people and what they mean to me – this thing called love. I'm in school and learning about relationships still. A song comes to mind; it's Michael Jackson singing, "*A-B-C, easy as 1-2-3, or simple as do-re-mi, Baby, you and me, gurl...*"

I realized and was reminded to sing to feel better. The vibrations of beats, the lines in the staff were homes to people. The notes: Mr. A is sharp and likes Mrs. B who is flat. Mr. A and Mr. B get married. They give birth to baby C. People were music to me with basic notes to basic beats.

I found humor with people, my music represented the people, now I was ready to face the music – grounded, protected and guided.

I could feel the dynamics, the drama of the collected friends in the backyard that Mike wanted me to meet or to help by coming to his emotional rescue. They were curious to meet me as Mike had described me to be a powerful psychic.

The usual questions were flowing: how I got this energy, what do I do with it, how could they benefit? One couple felt the energy come to them and a lift like a breath of fresh air. They thanked me for allowing them to feel love again. These people had lost their fortune and home to the casino and subsequently divorced. The ex-wife thanked me for allowing her ex-husband to feel compassion again – it was a good day for them.

There were other energy workers there who hadn't realized this was their destiny yet. They thanked me for my honesty and giving them courage to evolve in their journey.

I read the crowd and knew not everyone wanted to hear or were ready for the truth. I left the crowd, shut the conversations down and prepared to leave the party with Mike. The owner of the home had called me a satanist, said Mike. What was that, I thought? It reflected on the owner's own fears and energy, yet I respected her just the same. I wouldn't be accepted by some, though I did recognize the majority of the group was evolving to become aware and wanted more spiritual freedom.

Ironically that same night, Mike and I were gifted a 3,000 sq. ft. penthouse suite at the casino from the friend who lost everything to the casino. One night's complimentary stay was all he had left.

The next morning we ventured out to the darkest part of Detroit where Clint Eastwood was filming. This controversial film is about an older man who was very bigoted against the Chinese race. It will be a *Dirty Harry* movie where he breaks up the gang wars and saves the neighborhood in the end.

Homes were literally boarded up, glass laying on porches, lawns unkempt, tree debris left on the streets; these homes were valued at about $1,500. You wouldn't like to run out of gas in this part of Detroit. It was an ideal, ready-made set of a depressed neighborhood.

Security was tight. I could feel the calm and togetherness of the whole production – everything, I sensed, ran systematically and *very* smoothly with power and protection. It was a good feeling. I believe Clint commands this, and won't have anything less. The food trucks had traveled from California; the servers, the cooks, everything was coordinated for the production of eloquence. They all worked together to get the job done. Everyone served everyone's purpose to be there. These people were the best of the best, handpicked by the best with a clear purpose.

Mike was talking with Clint's longtime best friend from back in his Army days when I saw a tall man with a presence walking towards us… it was Clint.

He stopped, we were introduced, and he actually smiled and referred to me being another Canuck. *lol* We chatted and had a spiritual moment glance that seemed to last for minutes. He looked right into my eyes as if to read me – reading me with acceptance. Clint has presence and power to produce good things with meaning. A soulful purpose… he was granted power to survive the rest.

He went back in his trailer as the set had a break. I could feel his energy and felt he was getting and bringing in power, getting into position to deliver the next scene. He came out of the trailer keeping this energy in him and walked past us without conversation onto the set. He was in the zone….

He delivered the next scene and we broke for lunch.

Mike talked about the antioxidant food drink that I had brought with me. Clint wanted to know about it. I gave him a case of this special patented 19-fruit blend. He was interested and wanted to learn more... he took my card and website information. When the discussions were over we stood up and he took both of my hands, looked directly into my eyes and thanked me, saying it was a pleasure meeting you. He smiled and was off.

Talking to Mike the next day, Clint said he liked the juice as it gave him a kick of energy. He liked my smile and told Mike that I was a *keeper*.

I can *see* Clint looking at my card and being drawn to know more.... Or was that just the star-struck fan in me, thinking that? I will need powerful help if I'm to be educating the world, communicating on Clint's scale.

It was inspiring to see he was telling his stories (the movie messages), with a supporting cast and production company – all operating at the highest level without compromising his pursuit of quality and integrity. I too will need to assemble a manager and other helpers as I reach out to ever-increasing numbers of people, spreading my messages and building awareness.

MUSIC TRACK
Erasure asks for 'A Little Respect' and
why not listen to their 'Ship of Fools' also?
You know you're making me work so hard
... Soul, I hear you calling
Oh baby, please give a little respect to me.
Learning to respect yourself and setting boundaries.

CHAPTER 18

Cruisin' for a losin'

August 10 08, journal entry—

Two days later Mike and I were on a boat, meeting more new friends. We had been invited as guests on a cruise from Vancouver to Alaska.

The voyage to Alaska was both beautiful and ugly. It rained every day, with temperatures about 50 degrees. Cabin fever struck everybody. The aptly-named Inside Passage was a place to renew your soul – at the same time one could lose it. The people around were getting to me... at times I couldn't breathe. I needed to ground myself to help those good people around who needed me. There was always the buffet table... or a glass of wine. A slot machine perhaps. Let's get my nails done at the spa....

We sailed into Glacier Bay where we were only dozens of feet from layer upon layer of ice crystals formed tens of thousands of years ago. The bay was like a fjord enclosed by mountains. My heart and chest were beating with the vibrations that seemed to be bouncing back and forth off the mountains and fed by the ice and water. There was movement going on here! I could *feel* the Earth shifting and shaping into a new terrain. The mountains seem to hypnotize me. I couldn't move! Others were walking around the deck not paying much attention to what I could see, hear and feel. This was the best of the best healing energy I have ever felt on the west coast to date. I soaked it all in… that was the souvenir I would bring back home to others.

I noticed my mind was clear, I had a different perception to my own reality.

Then things started to crumble between Mike and I. He zigged and I zagged. I had to tell my truth, that I wanted more out of a relationship. He wanted out, I felt. I would go to sleep in our cabin; he wandered the halls of the ship at night. The next morning everyone knew Mike – he was a legend on the ship. (I would hate to see his bar tab at the end of the cruise.)

He forgot his high blood pressure pills. He had episodes of sweating, blacking out… no feeling in his limbs. I was apparently along to help him get through the trip. I let him make his choices. My mind was becoming clearer.

Mike wasn't feeling well. After healing him, I left him resting in the room. Ssshhhhh… Tiptoeing out… This third night would be my night!

High storm waves made my game of blackjack extra interesting. I remember looking at the dealer, pausing for an answer from up above whether to hit or not. He looked at me and said, "What are you, telepathic?"

I laughed to myself. The first card of my next hand was a 2. Before he dealt my second card, I paused, laughed and said, "I now have 6."

He looked at the card before giving it to me and said *you're freaking me out*. It was a 4.

I not only mastered the game between the dealer and myself, I could read the cards other players from China were playing (they didn't speak English). I learned how to control the table being the last draw card. Before long the Chinese were giving me *Hi-Fives. lol*

Would this give me a deeper soul? I certainly didn't need more shoes. I won a few thousand, then bought a couple of T-shirts and trinkets for my family back home. I bought nothing for me because I felt I really had everything I needed.

When I got back to the cabin, Mike had a stuffed puppy he had bought for me, flowers, and was waiting for me to come back to him. He waited for two hours, he said, and was unhappy that I was out. (Could this fella actually care more than I thought or was he just being selfish?)

We had a *come-to-Jesus* and got the truth out on the table. I was frightened and concerned that his learned behavior would burn him out. He was getting quite sick and I was exhausted healing him every night. We agreed to spend the next day together and try harder to get along.

When the ship docked at a small port, we were both ready and out of the cabin to go ashore shopping and sightseeing in the cold rain. Then Mike wanted to go back to the cabin (washroom break). He said he would meet me just off the boat ramp.

I waited and waited in the pouring rain. Finally I used my intuition to realize he wasn't coming. I went upstairs to the cabin... his hair was wet and he was changed into different clothing, no longer dressed for the wet weather. He was startled I'd came back and explained he went swimming and was coming down to meet me. *I lost it!* Changing into other clothing, I said I'd had *enough!*

I cried and cried knowing I didn't belong where I was at that moment, trying to release some of this energy and to get my own grounding back. I had no energy left to heal others let alone myself.

We spent some quiet time alone and I got back on my feet and was soon back healing and reading for others. My life seemed to be back to normal and as the cruise neared its end, I was determined to move on from Mike.

My friend Henry and his brother Nick were gracious to me. Not only had they bought me this first class ticket on the cruise, but they believed in me and wanted to work together in the near future. We first met in Hawaii while staying at Clint's house (Mike had arranged this). During an energy session then with Henry, I noticed spots on his liver and colon. I asked him to check this out with his doctor back home. It wasn't until months later that this issue I'd visualized showed up at a screening check-up with his doctor. Henry needed help – so from a distance we did two sessions prior to the cruise. Henry could feel the energy working exactly at the areas where I was sending it.

We were connecting for many reasons. Henry and Nick had another agenda for sponsoring me along on this cruise: they wanted me to help their longtime friend Mike from self-destructing. I told Henry it depends on Mike – on his desire to live in a positive environment within himself. We have given him the option. It was now up to him.

The trip ended with us coming into Georgia Strait towards Vancouver with the sun setting perfectly between two mountains and sinking into the sea. Picture orca whales breaching, dolphins dancing into the sun. A man had just proposed to his longtime girlfriend, tears and laughter were flowing from this estate cabin at the very back of the boat. Mike and I took a last sip of champagne from our respective glasses, looked at each other, made a wish and toasted the sea. *What will be, will be,* in our journeys. We toasted to peace between us for the rest of my stay.

Back in Vancouver Mike wanted to introduce me to his friend, who he calls his *Bro.* At dinner I was reading this fella. I've met many dangerous men in my life, but not like this one. This one was for hire – and not to change a flat tire on your car. He was a highly-trained martial arts and guns expert who hurts people for a living! I could see into his eyes and tell you why, what went wrong, his life's influences, why he couldn't help himself. Mike did warn me that he has no conscience and was a ruthless killer, but I'd assumed Mike had been exaggerating until now.

I wanted the truth. Why did these two called each other *Bro?* How often did they see each other? I realized it didn't matter. Mike could read me!

We were sitting on a patio and Mike's friend was squishing spiders that would fall close to my head. A little foreshadowing? Why was I meant to meet this guy? My mind was racing. Why was I meant to meet so many people like this over my lifetime? He wasn't the first hit man who has walked into my path. I knew that other people would only see these people in the movies or hear about them through others.

Mike disappeared into the restaurant next door to his condo. I could *see* from afar that he was flirting with a redhead. After hearing one too many horror story from Mike's friend, I got up to verify Mike's disappearance. Sure enough he was sitting at a table getting cozy with a young female with red hair. I left the restaurant, feeling dizzy and hurt.

I immediately called to book the very next flight back home.

Mike apologized *for my reaction*. He denied the girl thingy but admitted he needed to distance himself from the dark side. He asked me why he did such a thing.

To scare me away and for you to see what you can't see, I told him. He agreed and was sorry. He begged me to stay and have one more peaceful day together – he wanted to learn more from me.

As a healer, was I the one he would listen to? My mind was made up regardless. Healthy boundaries were necessary for me. I was tired of healing: it was time to go home.

On the way to the airport, Mike wanted to clear a few things up. He was thanking me for bringing awareness to him that he couldn't see before.

"Yes," he replied bitterly, "the redhead likes me and you could see *that*."

He was insulting my intelligence again, and my patience had worn out. Normally I would respect anyone's awareness and say nothing, but this guy was getting under my skin.

"She's young enough to be your daughter and you are searching for love in all the wrong places," I told him. "You're looking for acceptance – but you've got to find the love *inside yourself*."

He promised he would stop his drinking during the week. He wanted to make it right….

This conversation only minutes to the airport was going nowhere. He walked me to Departures. I said goodbye and turned the corner. I couldn't help this man. He needed to help himself. My angels had said this will be a good day. So who needs angels anyway? *Sigh.*

Two days later, Mike called and left a message as if he was the captain from the boat, leaving his funny Irish stories, something about the history of the donut. *lol* He said that since I left him the pain was terrible in his back and he wanted to fly me back to Vancouver or he was coming to Ontario for a fix. Hhhmmm. What could be causing that pain?

MUSIC TRACK
Hear Weezer's 'Island In The Sun'
I can't control my brain
… We'll spend some time forever
We'll never feel bad anymore
A great vibey, visually-stimulating song with warm imagery to
think about. You can actually feel it without controlling the brain.
Excellent to raise your vibrations for that warm fuzzy feelin'
(listen for the cool guitar lick).

CHAPTER 19

My first healing session from Sharon

ugust 23 08, journal entry—
I remember getting ready at home and feeling heat, my breathing was more intense. It was Sharon, our energies were connecting already – this would be my first energy session as her client! I was excited and couldn't wait to get rid of some of the heaviness I was feeling after the cruise. My goal was to be so light and airy I could concentrate better on what I needed to do for myself instead of concentrating on other people's issues.

I purposely made up my eyes to be a darker shade of brown, trying to mask the golden yellow brown eyes that are so similar to Sharon's. I did this to make Sharon at ease so that she could look at me. Some people had told me they couldn't look into my eyes – the eyes seemed to draw them in as if I was looking right through them.

Sharon answered her door (with her knitting in hand) with *those eyes* that pulled me in to accepting her energy. Her home was decorated similar to mine, with earthy tones, comfy couches, paintings of intriguing ladies, some accent furniture made to look warm, gothic mirrors, landscape pictures of flowers and trees, candles burning, and the photos of doors we both adore that remind us of portals. I felt at home.

In her basement was a room appointed with cleansing rock salts, candles and incense. The vibrations I could feel were high in this protected room. I knew she had the gift. It was an interesting massage, not like I had experienced before. She closes her eyes to work (much like I do) and feels where the energy is. Her hands lead her to the spots to push on. A rose quartz was placed on my belly. As I laid on my back, Sharon would put her hands underneath my body and place her fingers to push on spots between my shoulder blades. My tummy started rumbling and moving intensely, the energy filling the rose quartz crystal. The energy I was storing was others' energy. I'd been carrying other people's stuff. It was all coming out – past life and this life!

Sharon said there is a person standing at my head. This 4-foot 5-inch lady figure had a message for me. Sharon saw and heard the name of this figure to be Anna. Anna had a stick in her hand and was not pleased with my friend Mike. Anna was showing me that if I am to build a pyramid with sticks, this stick of Mike doesn't fit into my pyramid. It only slows the process down. Anna was telling me to keep on my path of less destruction.

I would have to define this relationship, so I asked for direction. Anna said I gave more of my energy to him than he could offer to me. There was light and dark in everyone. His light side is very good. However you must know that this dark side in him comes with him forever. That is who he is. He is the whole package. When you leave him, he is in pain as the dark side is trying to claw back. Hence the pain in his back.

Sharon and I were sharing visuals – we knew we would work together. I saw her traveling with me to other countries, the southern US west coast to be specific. England, Caribbean… We didn't know how or what, we simply accepted what the angels were showing us at this time. Sharon wanted to council me, guide me to what I couldn't see, and be a protector as well. She saw me being in the forefront… two sisters dancing with laughter and playing with the energy, helping people around the world.

I left her home. The last thing she said, "You look just like me. I can't look at you." *lol*

Yes, we laughed out loud quite heartily.

When I got home, the energy was so strong that my dog Cubo for the first time didn't sleep on my bed. He was up all night chasing spirits through the house, barking as if someone was there. The visions and dreams took me to many planes: I could see the future, I was getting messages of warning – I was in the loop!

Trance-like, Cubo and I slept most of the next day.

I was healing. I was rebooting. I was renewing my soul.

MUSIC TRACK
[requested by Gabrielle]:
General Public performing 'Tenderness'
Searching for it
… where is it?
… I held your hand

CHAPTER 20

Gabrielle's advice

An email from Donna and Gabrielle came the morning after my session with Sharon, with affirmation to all the questions I had. Precisely when I needed it.

Donna usually loses herself to Gabrielle partway through an email. When she starts writing an email, usually she doesn't know why – until she presses the *send* button and looks back at what was typed. We both have in common that we can't usually remember everything in angel talk. That is because there is a lot of detail and generally it's not our stuff. It's for others to retain, not us.

Donna can speak on and on for hours, it seems, as a conduit for Gabrielle. Sometimes when we are face-to-face, she'll say, "Okay, Nadine, pull me out. I can't get out of the trance or vibrations."

Donna writing in an email—

Good Morning, Nadine!

It's been ages since I've caught up with you! How was the cruise? I can only imagine that it was absolutely incredible!

These summer months have flown by. I had to really focus on making money this summer, and the focus has paid off – priority seemed to be the lesson of the day. *lol*

It's been a summer of helping people it seems. So many people who are bored and sad, all for different reasons. It's been difficult to fill in the gaps with everyone. And most of the time, the gap is simply laughter. *lol*

Laughter and direction, peace and love, compassion and understanding... we all need so much more of that. Imagine: if everyone had more of a smile on their face, you may not have emotionally sick people to heal! *lol*

I kind of went into hibernation in July because I couldn't process, or better yet, seem to get a grip on some form of negativity that kept engulfing my space. No one around me seemed to be happy and it was extremely draining. I just started to chill and focus on working and trying to earn much-needed money. That aspect of my life is a necessity.

Gabrielle speaking through Donna—

We are not alone on these ships that we travel through life on. We are in the company of friends, family, acquaintances and co-workers. We're not suppose to get away from these people, however we are suppose to get organized, otherwise our ship will be in complete chaos. And it may even get so imbalanced that it feels like it's sinking.

Finding our particular balance is paramount – and it's much more productive to take a few minutes, or hours, or days, or even months, to re-balance ourselves and resume our post, rather than get so imbalanced that we forget our direction completely, never to resume or accomplish our ultimate life contract.

Happiness, goodness and purity of heart will conquer all. The darkest of individuals can be lightened with just a bit of sugar – but it's not that the sugar will change them, it just makes them easier for those around to tolerate. Just like sugar in coffee; it only sweetens the cup, not the whole pot!

Realizing exactly where we fit in on our boat is not difficult. We are the captains. We are all the captains of our own ships.

Balance, balance, balance... understanding, understanding, understanding... and the clear knowledge that all is well and will proceed at a course of abundance as soon as we get our ship properly loaded and balanced. Then the waters will be easy to navigate, regardless of the conditions. Our path will be so much easier!

It is stated, "On Earth as it is in Heaven." The tranquility, power and peace of the Universe is there for all to have on Earth. Mankind has made its own kind of Hell, thriving on hatred, contempt, jealousy, greed and lust. That's the recipe for death – not physical, but spiritual. All inhabitants of Earth are born into the physical plane with a spiritual tie to the Universe. Some lose the connection, just like losing radio contact. Others develop booster stations, to make the connection stronger and clearer. The disconnected can be guided or instructed to retune their radios... but they cannot be forced, they must use their own power from within.

With the light you go... and with the power of the light you must travel, just like a missionary in a foreign country. It is with the power of the Universe that goodness will come, sugar will be provided for the dark, bitter coffee, and the lights around you will only become brighter. The ship will be balanced as you chart your course.

With love and peace,

Shurean, Gabrielle et al

Shurean? Another angel or guide? Guess I need all the angels I can get. I need angels! Please send me more angels.

I'm writing these passages about waters and the need to balance your ship. Mike calls to say he is happy and in a better state of mind, despite that it's pouring rain and his boat that he just got fixed is sinking at the marina. (What are the chances?)

I read him Donna's writing from the angels. He was blown away like the fog horn blows when you can't see in the fog, warning other ships in his path. (Cheesy, corny, but true.) *lol*

"This is the captain of the boat speaking. It's a fine sunny day. There's room for everyone on this journey to make the right choices to keep your boat afloat with laughter."

Why am I letting this guy slide his way back into my life?

Relayed by Donna—

The message in your cards is that you're on assignment for the Higher Power, and it's a path that will be humbling on one hand, yet extremely rich on the other. Faith, pure faith is so important. It's not about all the Earthly riches that you've become accustomed to – and even worshipped at times, it's about something much larger and something on a much more global theme. The Holy Spirit is with you, The Force as some may call it, and will continuously direct you where you have to be. You must once and for all let go of unwanted patterns – whether they be thought processes, concerns and/or relationships. Just simply cast them away as if they were finished chapters in a book. It takes time and energy to put things into order, and there never seems to be enough hours in the day, so ask us to do it for you. Have faith that we will make the path much easier for you. Your partners must have faith in our work – it is not a circus act, and it must be done as according to the divine plan... we will clear your path.

Ask us for help. You know we cannot help unless asked. Unless you're getting run over by a bus or something – and even then we really shouldn't step in – you must ask. You have megawatts of energy emanating from your soul and it only stands to reason that many have tapped into it. Clear the fat off of the belly of the pig. There is no right. There is no wrong. But there are those with ulterior motives, agendas that don't quite match your purpose, and it may take you months if not years to deal with them. Ask us and we will clear the path immediately.

Just ask – there are a lot of us looking over you.

Email from Donna—

I've been feeling compelled to pick up a tarot deck and an Angel deck of cards. I tossed out a few Angel cards for you tonight – I think it's important stuff.

Archangel Michael is with you, and has been with you as a guiding force, protecting you and providing you wisdom to make sure you are safe and can complete your tasks without worry.

St. Mother Teresa is with you, providing you the wisdom to reach out to those in need with compassion, humility and understanding.

St. Agnes of Rome is with you, under the *Don't Compromise* card. Do not give in to intimidation or luring to sacrifice your integrity or morals. You have important work to do and are being protected by God. Expand yourself without concern for those who want to rape you, because they can't get near you. Don't do something until it's 100% correct with you!

Your Guardian Angel is providing you *Blessings of Abundance*. You will not be let down. You shall receive what you need. Your Guardian Angel is giving you the foresight of a child – the clear, undiluted thoughts. Thoughts that will not be tainted with the knowledge of years gone by, but an innocence that all is pure and blessed from this day forward.

Listen to Wallflowers play 'One Headlight'
But there's got to be an opening
Somewhere here in front of me
Through this maze of ugliness and greed
... Hey, come on try a little
Nothing is forever
A little vibey rock song about losing a friend to disease,
listening in silence, wondering.

CHAPTER 21

Results

August 23 08, journal entry—

Roy called to inform me that he just had a meeting with his oncologist. According to a CT scan there was nothing on his liver to indicate a tumor – the cancer is gone.

A CT scan is a series of x-rays taken from different angles as the body is passed through the scanner and exposed to radiation. This produces a 3-dimensional view of the body and highlights any imperfections.

To recap the sequence of events: Roy was diagnosed with colorectal cancer in June of 2003 which had also spread to his liver. So he underwent colon surgery on June 21st and a 70% liver resection on September 09, 2003. Roy was cancer free for three and a half years when his CEA (carcinoembryonic antigen, the tumor markers in his blood) levels began to elevate. In December of 2006 he was diagnosed with a 20 cm tumor on the old part of his liver (cells probably there but not active or detectable during first surgery) and it resided next to the only artery left feeding his liver. Chemotherapy began in January

2007. After sixteen months of chemo and several MRIs (magnetic resonance imaging) to monitor the size of the tumor, the last one being on April 09, 2008, it still was not shrinking. On April 14, 2008 he met with his liver surgeon who reported the tumor, at the size it was and not appearing to shrink any further with the chemo treatments, was too large and too close to the artery; the surgeon didn't think he could ever operate without putting Roy's life in extreme danger. Roy and I had our first energy session on April 22 of 2007. In late June, he began taking the drug Erbitux. Now in late August, the CT scans are showing *nothing* on the liver and the CEA levels in his blood have been down to a normal range since June. Meanwhile, my readings are urging that detoxification of the body is necessary to complete the healing process.

Dr. Diana (Roy's naturopathic doctor) will be coming this week to experience a session. Dr. Diana is now referring his clients with tumors to me based on his studies with Roy and myself. He told me he had more visions of waving his hands naturally over his client's body and the disease would disappear. He didn't understand his visions but now believes he has this in him to help in the same manner as I do. I will teach Dr. Diana what I know.

⁓❧

24 August 08, journal entry—

A few months ago, I was talking on the phone with a salesman who was trying to sell me Internet advertising space to attract people to a website I was building. As I was asking questions, automatically Jessie started receiving my energy. He was in California; I was in Ontario, Canada. He instantly felt the energy and was amazed to the point he felt different and was telling people in his office what had just happened. His pain had disappeared, he could think more clearly. The co-workers couldn't believe it so I began freely sending energy over the phone to several of his co-workers and family members for the remainder of the day and evening.

Later he reported they *all* felt the energy and claimed to be changed people. Jessie thanked me for making them believers and said that he needed to be a part of building awareness. Jessie wanted the world to know, and offered to help with my website promotions without charge. Like Clint and his filming, I'll need excellent production help – here's an expert volunteering his services.

Jessie called the very evening my new healer friend Sharon was getting to know me. He spoke to Sharon, giving her validation that the energy healing exists from a distance as well. He could feel the energy of the two of us. It was strong, he said.

⚓

3 September 08, incoming testimonial emails—

I was in the throws of a major health scare – I needed to calm down, stop thinking worst case scenario, and get a little perspective. A friend who's a psychotherapist told me about Nadine and maybe she could help me. I knew nothing about Nadine, only that my friend thought she was the *real deal*. Well, in the shape I was in, I was willing to try anything, and I wasn't disappointed. I'm about as down to Earth as you can get, and in the time I spent with Nadine I was nothing short of wowed. After a brief session/energy healing, not only were my spirits lifted, but my back pain (which has nothing to do with why I went) was alleviated. How? I have no idea, but one thing I'm sure about is that she is the *real deal*.

Thank you, Nadine!

– Danielle

I was referred to Nadine by a colleague of mine who is probably one of the biggest skeptics I know! I had a car accident in May 2007, a lot of soft tissue damage in my back, shoulders and neck. The accident also triggered my TMJ (temporo-mandibular joint), which I had surgery for in 1997. Since this surgery I have had nerve damage and no feeling in the left side of my face.

During my first telephone conversation with Nadine, we talked for quite a while and I set up an appointment with her. I did not tell her about my TMJ – basically I told her I feel that I have lost focus, energy, and was sick of going from one doctor to another.

The next morning after our conversation, I got up, did my morning thing: coffee, paper, etc. and all of sudden noticed that I had full feeling in the left side of my face!

I also had been going to the dentist once a week to try and adjust my jaw. We try weekly to get one millimeter or so more open than the previous week. My dentist was absolutely astonished that in one week I had over 10 millimeters increased movement in my jaw, no more pain, etc. Nadine and I had not even discussed distance healing until my upcoming visit.

I then had my actual appointment with Nadine after all of this which was utterly profound. My energy level, my optimism, my sense of calm, which were things I was really concerned with, are just wonderful.

It is difficult to explain how differently I feel. My accident problems are literally gone. I am off all the meds from the accident. Emotionally, I have not felt this in control and calm in many years.

I have referred numerous people to Nadine. She is truly genuine, an angel who will give her heart and soul to people in need of physical and mental well-being.

God Bless and thank you, Nadine.

Regards,

– Sue

A woman (call her "A") tried to commit suicide by overdosing on drugs while in Africa. Paul was called to heal her from Vancouver but had difficulty reading the situation. Adam was in Poland at the time. With Paul and I working together, it took all of 15 minutes to send and for A to receive the energy to get this result below to save her life.

Dear Paul,

A is doing so much better today. Her liver enzyme level dropped from 800 (when we started to heal her) to 300 (today). Normal level should be around 40. So it is coming.

Also, she started to eat a little bit today.

I think she will be OK.

Please accept my gratitude for helping her. Please let Nadine know also my gratitude.

Thank you,

– Adam

I was referred to Nadine Mercey by a friend and never so glad to receive a suggestion. I started to see her in September/07.

My emotional well-being could best be described as a roller coaster ride and was way off. Over the years I had accumulated several diagnoses including chronic depression, generalized anxiety disorder and Attention Deficit Disorder. I was on the maximum medication for these. I also have carpal tunnel, chronic neck pain, osteoarthritis, elevated cholesterol, gastroesophageal reflux and a variety of other aches and pains. My home life was chaotic.

Within three visits with Nadine my neck pain was gone. I had more energy and was not so easily upset. My self-esteem began to rise and I started to wean off of my medications (under a physician's care). My concentration and memory began to return. My heartburn vanished and the remaining symptoms significantly decreased.

By December/07 I was off all medications and I continue to improve. I cannot say enough about Nadine, particularly concerning her approachability, kindness and empathy. Her healing abilities are profound. Not a day goes by that I don't thank the 'Powers That Be' for bringing her into my life.

– Jill C

When writing a testimonial I suppose it's important to think about the intended audience. Should I write this for curious skeptics, or for believers?

Well, it really doesn't matter because I walked in a skeptic and came out a believer. Nadine is a healer of both body and spirit – and she radiates positive energy and it's impossible to not feel better after a session with her.

Thank you so much,

– Danielle

To Those of You About To Change Your Life,

Here is my story:

In 2006, I began to feel very tired and run down. This feeling grew and grew until I desperately began seeking help through the normal channels of our health care. They first discovered that I had no vitamin

B12 in my body (not at all normal for a woman my age) and began to treat me accordingly. They counseled me to reduce my stress level, as that was the likely culprit. But by early 2007, I knew I was in trouble. My fatigue grew increasingly worse. I was plagued with pain throughout my body. My joints were growing increasingly stiff and movement was becoming more and more difficult.

In March 2007, I came down with a fever of 104°F, which lasted for 5 weeks. I nearly lost my eyesight to a disease called iritis (a disease caused by severe swelling of the eye's iris tissues which is indicative of a complete organ failure at the severe degree I had it). Finally, my situation was deemed serious enough to gain some attention and my journey through a long line of specialists and doctors began.

By December of 2007, being self-employed, I felt defeated and was heading into financial ruin. I was exhausted from the time I woke in the morning and the pain was spreading throughout my body. Despite all of my desperate attempts I still had no answers from the medical profession other than I was very sick and they did not know why. The medications they had me on to control the inflammation and other symptoms had warnings 10 to 20 pages long and seemed to be killing me a little quicker than the disease itself. One of the medications alone was going to cost me $22,000/year!

Lucky for me, my boss had seen Nadine a few weeks before and urged me to see her too. He indicated he had been skeptical, but had indeed received freedom for the pain of his herniated disks as he had requested her to do. He seemed shocked, amazed and relieved that finally he had his life back and that he would not require surgery after all, and the journey for healing had come full circle for him.

So, financially destitute as I was at the time, I was desperate and truly felt my life was coming to a close. Being a single mom, this was a very difficult thing for me to accept. So, I called Nadine, set up the appointment with hopes that somehow she could give me enough of *something* to at least keep me holding on until the doctors could help me.

Indeed, what I received from her was a gift of complete and total healing. No more pain, no more problems with my eyesight, no more debilitating cramps in my muscles, no more fatigue. The day I brought Nadine into my life, was the day I received my life back in full color, free from the burdens of my past. Free to explore all of the opportunities that life has since presented to me in a major way.

Today, just three weeks after first meeting Nadine, I am a new person, both spiritually and physically. Thank you, Nadine. You have changed my life and, since then, the lives of many people that those you have helped, have referred your way! You go, girl. Heal this world... one person at a time, even if we don't know it... we need you!!!!

If you are considering if this may be for you, STOP wondering. It is for you. In fact it is a shame that Nadine cannot be there for us all. Make no mistake, you need to take action now. Pick up the phone and call her. For your own sake, don't wait, run!!!!

Sincerely,

– Karen D

Dearest Nadine, I cannot thank you enough for Wed. I do feel very different. In some ways I can't explain. In others... I feel lighter. I feel more protected like the Sun is by my side and protecting my heart at all times. On the day of our session at one point I could see the Sun going into my body and healing certain areas. The pain you worked on was greatly, greatly reduced and still reducing. I did a healing session on myself this morning. I think it went pretty well I even got 5 or 6 burps out. Thank you so so much for your love, compassion and healing. Thanks for teaching and sharing with me. Thank you for getting me closer to achieving my goals and dreams. Thanks for helping me be myself.

Take care

Love, Peace and successful book grease!

– Katie

MUSIC TRACK
Ronan Keating plays 'Lovin' Each Day'
We're loving each day as if it's the last
Dancing all night and havin' a blast
… So don't go throwing our love away
It's here to stay

CHAPTER 22

A day in the life

What's it like being a psychic and a healer?

Casino runs are fun. JACKPOTS!!!

When I ask *inside* and get an okay to make some money, it can be a lot of fun. Usually I just play the slots because that's all I need. I believe in being respectful and only taking home what I need for a particular project or purpose. It's very difficult to be in the money vibration of ego with others for very long when you're a healer.

I don't allow my 16-year-old son to play for money. He reads and can tell you what cards people are holding.

Being a healer and psychic mom, my abilities can be helpful to know when their homework isn't done, what issues they are having. Communication is wonderful with my Eric and Jaxon. They have matured nicely. So I advise people to develop your intuition not only to be more physically healthy: it's great for family relationships too!

As you might guess, dating has been interesting.

Dialing it up and down is interesting – I can make my energy change

168

when going into a new situation or when building rapport with new faces – very useful in real estate work but sometimes misunderstood in social settings.

My friend (Prince Harming) would say he'd dated some pretty good-looking women who turn heads, but he had a hard time dealing with the attention or looks I got. I impressed, I explained, because their souls were meeting with mine – it wasn't the skirt or the hair, honey. It's about my higher purpose raising soul vibrations.

On the other hand, a high level positive vibration keeps away what I call the *Takers* with adverse energies, because like energies attract and dissimilar ones repel each other.

⁂

4 September 08, journal entry—

Last week I was called to study the energy of an 180-year-old house that had been renovated and fixed up to sell. The vendors haven't been able to secure a buyer despite many market pluses. This home has curb appeal. It was well priced with a very good agent and a reputable company representing it.

When I walked into the home, there was a sense of familiarity to it. I was comfortable in parts of the home but not others. The kitchen I could sense needed help in the electricals. I sensed the fan needed work and opened up a cupboard to point out a central location of adverse energy which happened to be in the electric control panel of the home. The listing agent was surprised to find the electrical panel in there. In my experience the energies love to play havoc with the electrical system – their vibrations resonate there.

The office was perfect. I could breathe and stay there for a long time...

The master bedroom was horrid!!! Burp burp burp. I had to clear the energy in the room. The ensuite next to it was fine.

The basement is where most of the energy laid (unrested). Apparently, according to history books, this home was a link in the *underground railway system* where enlightened white folks brought slaves from the USA to hide almost 200 years ago.

I cleared the energy and freed the vibrations there (it was from many, many souls ago). I was tired but went back through the house to double-check and found all was at peace there. My job was done.

Over lunchtime (and wanting some deserved rest) I walked into only two shops….

The first was a bath shop (how relaxing, I thought). The owner of the store had lost her hair and a breast to cancer. Not wanting to consciously try to clear her toxic energy from the medications I stepped away and looked at soaps in a corner. My body started to heat up. Yup, I couldn't breathe. The energy clearing process was starting and I soon would be burping out loud in a public store.

Noel, the owner, came up to me and said, "It's cool if you're a healer. My boyfriend can sense things too. I understand. There's the sink if you need it."

I thought to myself: in Ontario we wouldn't be having these conversations in public a few years ago. My, how the world has progressed while I had been hiding and not aware myself.

Normally the energy isn't that strong where it takes over my personal time. I wondered maybe Noel was an important link in my future process for this meeting to take place? Only time will tell.

Now what trouble could I get into in the next store – a women's fine tailored dress store?

As I walked in, the owner of the store at that very moment by coincidence (hhhhmmm) remarked that she was in severe pain with Bell's palsy.

"Oh no, not again, so fast," I thought. "I haven't had time to rejuvenate."

Kathyrn was her name (I recalled a message from a few days prior that a Kathryn would want my help). She gave me a couple of outfits to try on in the dressing room.

Yup. I was heating up and deep breathing. The energy exchange was taking place and Kathryn was possibly 50 feet away from me. Burp, burp, burp.

"Ugh, ugh, ugh," I thought. "Not now in this fine establishment – in a change room? What will the young assistant think as she does the pinning and helping with alterations?"

Just then Kathryn explained to the young girl that I was a healer, and am clearing the pain away to help her.

The young girl replied, "That's so cool. I've got a singing part in the musical *Age of Aquarious.*"

lol How appropriate.

Soon Kathryn's pain was gone and that was all that mattered. Then I relayed important messages for Kathryn that came through for her betterment and awareness. She was grateful and gave me a discount on a scarf for being a kindred spirit.

Next she gave me a business card of a psychic reader who she felt I needed to connect with....

Now I know what you're thinking: How could anyone take Nadine out to a fine restaurant with all this burping happening?

I can and I have been able to control the spontaneous energy events to a point. Sometimes, however, I do need to excuse myself and clear the energy while in a restroom or outside on a patio. Usually I am protected so this doesn't interfere with my personal life.

One of the most rewarding things for me are the little conversations (the random meetings) I have with people who have quite limited knowledge about the energy or the bigger picture. I love to talk to those who are looking for answers but don't know they are looking. [If that makes sense – I just happen to fall into their path by so-called coincidence and make an impact that sticks!]

This week, one of my goals was to contact a supplier for the detox bath product line we are developing. I phoned one of the many sources, picking at random.

The manager spends 90 minutes on the phone talking to me about the whys, hows and whats of my energy knowledge. Finally he admits that throughout our lengthy conversation, he was feeling guilty about not spending time having a coffee with his own mother who is suffering with cancer. Why did he spend so long talking over the phone to a stranger instead of devoting that time with his own mother?

What he hadn't known was that while he was feeling guilty, I had been directing energy to him. This gentleman was grateful that I reduced his fears so that he could be stronger to deal with his mother who needed him. This man will now pay it forward to his mother and give her the strength she needs at this pivotal time.

He asked if he could pay me for my time.

"If we would just stop to take the time to help others when we could," I told him, "the Universe would look after things and it will all work out to benefit us all. This healing was for free. Pass it on."

Then I got an email from a social worker who was organizing an awareness fair for teachers. Would I come and be a guest speaker? I asked myself where did this come from? Turns out to be a suggestion to her from someone I'd randomly helped only last week. *lol*

Open-minded people aren't afraid of *random* meetings – because they know people are sent to them for a reason, just when they need them. So nothing is truly random – it's simply an opportunity you seize or pass by.

Donna had a funny *random* meeting the other day. She was in a drive-thru line of about 10 cars. A lady knocks on her window (of all the cars) and asks if Donna knows where a certain address was. Donna says that if she jumps in the car it would be only a few minutes drive to her destination. This lady doesn't own a car – she'd come by bus. Donna feels compelled to buy her a coffee and to drive her to the destination. (I know Donna. *lol* She's thinking: wow, like this could be Mary Magdalene or Jesus in disguise. *lol* Most people would be afraid of bringing strangers into their cars!) Donna drives her to the right street but the address doesn't exist! Donna brings her back to Tim Horton's and enjoyed the energy and the conversation. The lady who arrived by bus was then off on her way. Hhhhmmmm...

Maybe not Mary or Jesus. Perhaps one of his twelve disciples in drag, eh, Donna? *lol*

MUSIC TRACK
Pete Townsend rocking through 'Let My Love Open the Door'
When everything feels all over
When everybody seems unkind
It sometimes takes others to make you see, to give you hope
for your own self-worth. Just when you need them,
it's your lucky day – or is it fate?

CHAPTER 23

The angels explain

September 15 08, journal entry with emails—

Donna and I asked some questions of the angels and received some pretty bright responses which I've written out below. This does resonate with me – it's just hard for me to translate into written English. Donna did a great job! I hear the humor as the angels make me laugh all day long just as Donna puts it below in writing. They are hilarious.

We asked about who all the angels were because some of them gave themselves names when they communicated with us. We added Abraham to the list because two nights ago a voice came into my mind, identified itself as Abraham and mentioned upcoming work I needed to do. It was so clear at the time, I thought I would remember and didn't write down the specifics. We were having lovely conversations. He wants to help our work. Then yesterday someone bought me a ticket and suggested I needed to go to see the upcoming Abraham-Hicks seminar in Toronto. The Hicks (Jerry and Esther, a husband and wife team) channel a guide called Abraham! Abraham-Hicks wrote *The Law of Attraction*, the book that has inspired millions, been adapted by dozens of other authors and is the focus of *The Secret*.

Donna emailed: I just picked up your e-mail... yes... it's 6:27 am... I am studying... lol... since 5 am... lol

I do have a message for you which will clarify things... I believe! [Donna's email continues as the angels, who refer to themselves as Gabrielle et al, dictate to her—]

Good Morning, Nadine,

So many questions!!!! Sometimes it is with great difficulty that we're able to explain in words certain things that are truly vibrational in nature, however, we will give you the clearest picture possible, so it can be understood and absorbed.

Many months ago, you were guided to raise the vibrational level of Donna. You were advised that she was to be awakened and brought to a level of consciousness that would allow this communication. We thank you.

We are a collective universal body or consciousness, shall we say. We are what would be perceived in Earthly terms as a feminine energy, or wisdom chamber, from which all on Earth can learn. We are neither female or male, however, our lessons to mankind bear teachings of what would be considered Earthly feminine traits, that being the love of a mother, the compassion of a sister and the beauty and innocence of a little girl, combined with the wisdom of the Universal One, which is always perceived to be a more masculine energy. The protector, the wise one. We are a collective, and we are here to guide you in guiding just as we are here to guide many. We are very much part of Abraham, the Echo and all heavenly guidance systems.

There is always a desire to confuse the issue of where divine information comes from. If it's not from God, then many believe that it is from the darker side of the cube. However, this is not the case, at all. We are not one particular angel, we are not one particular saint, we are not one particular body, we are a collective. On our vibrational plane, our plane of existence, perception from an Earthly realm is not possible. We don't exist within your level of perception, however, our vibrational characteristics make it entirely possible for you to feel us and sense us. We are wisdoms and energies forever drawing on the Source and the archangels whose energies can be called upon and tapped into at any time, for they are all powerful, graced with this ability from the Universal One, or God, or the Higher Power.

It always seems to be a necessity that mankind adopts a particular angel. However all the archangels are there, with everyone, every day of life. In saying that we must clarify, that it is not a particular angel, but the energies of all of the angels for the asking. All one has to do is believe, all one has to do is have faith. Those who believe will benefit greatly in their faith and trust.

We are a collective of wisdom. We are a guidance system. Gabrielle is our name. We are not tied into one particular angel or saint, as none of those that we address are tied into any one particular angel or saint. You do have energies that you tap into more one day than another, but all is guided supremely by the context and depth of your faith and belief that particular day.

Now, the question which many have, and that is: Why? Why now?... Well, the answer is quite simple. We have always been, and we have always spoke, however we have not always been heard. A few have heard and followed, and have had faith that their beliefs were right and have actually lost their Earthly lives for such a belief. This was not the intent of our teachings. It has taken much time on the Earthly plane to understand that the Universal One is an all-loving God. And that the Universal One is all passionate and all forgiving. The Universal One is all loving. Evil is manmade, a condition of the Ego, while goodness is the birthright of the Soul.

For even those who do not believe in an existence beyond Earthly death, there is grace and forgiveness. For even those who cause hardship, there is grace and forgiveness. However, the path that their energy takes will be totally different than the paths of those energies or souls that truly live in an elevated state of consciousness.

Our collective is here to spread the news to all who can hear and can listen. It is a very logical collective, just as the Abraham Collective is logical. It is the path to an elevated spirituality, an elevated faith, an elevated belief.

You have never been alone. Why is it that a lion never thinks about the last chunk of venison that he wolfed down and why is it that many people of an enlightened nature feel mortified when they strike a bunny rabbit with their car? Why is it that people of Christian background feel great re-morse upon taking the life of another man, when others feel it is their ob-ligation or right? Believe us when we say that absolutely no one from the higher power would give authority to anyone by way of religion to take the life of another man. There is no difference between taking the life of a physical man, woman or child. They are all lives, they are all souls. We are here to help all those who can hear to raise the vibrational levels of good-ness and grace. Powers that can move mountains and still waters. Powers that can stop wars and move the Earth forward to peace and love.

The marriage between body and soul is awe inspiring. It is a creation of great, unbelievable proportions.

Many current day energies have been part of our collective, and have chosen for their own growth to rebound to the Earthly plane. You can picture us as thousands of professors sitting around a huge table, but we are simply a huge mass of energies. Yes, Man was created in the image of God, but we are not man. We are a force of the Universal One, available to you in whatever form you desire us to be in.

"Let there be Peace on Earth." Let there be love, truth, faith and un-derstanding. Let there be forgiveness on every level.

For all things are possible. Yes. All things are possible. Manifesting is simply an equation. Belief + faith + desire = manifestation. The higher the vibrations of mankind, the easier this equation will be, and yes, this simple mathematical equation can make peace on earth. It can end war, end weather catastrophes and end starvation. The power is in mankind to change the surroundings that mankind must live in. It can truly be Heaven on Earth.

The teachings of Abraham and various other Believe-and-you-shall-receive teachings serve to raise many vibrations. Once man sees, he be-comes a believer, develops more faith, thus more desire, thus better mani-festations. All things are possible.

In closing, we trust that you will find the wisdom in our words. We trust that your heart will be lighter by all that we say. We trust that you will understand who we are and why we are here. We are to be known as Gabrielle, or the Gabrielle Collective, or the Gabrielle Clan, whatever is easiest for you. We are here with Donna and many others. Donna's energies have existed with Gabrielle, as have many energies around her.

She has always been in communication with the collective, as have many around her. Here is where her wisdom has come from. She has neither been chosen nor created abilities, she has simply always been connected and has connected with those of correct vibrational frequencies.

On occasion, particular energies take the podium, so to speak. It's more like an exclamation mark. The energies of that particular energy may be referred to, but the name will only have coincidental meaning. Teresa, Joan, Harry, John... they're simply names separating the collective from one particular energy, with thoughts of a masculine or feminine nature. The Angels of the Higher Power do not give us any sticky notes to pass on to anyone. All must have faith in their existence, as all must have faith in the Higher Power, and ask for their guidance. We cannot forgive you, we cannot save you from a perceived Hell, but we can give you the wisdom and the knowledge to make all things possible.

We act in the highest and best service to the Universal One, for now and forever.

Gabrielle et al

⚬

16 September 08, more messages from Gabrielle et al—

Abraham is not being channeled to Esther Hicks. She knows she came here with that information. She speaks with them as one. Esther is not speaking apart from Abraham. We label things for what we perceive.

Energy came in to awaken Esther just as Donna was awaken by Nadine to remember. To heighten vibration is to return to a state where you have been before awakening, that has always been with you. Living on the Earthly plane, you can't grow if you have to remember everything without being reborn or refreshed.

⚬

Donna and I go into trance, going in and out of a state of consciousness, into a different spot to block out visual stimuli (such as closing your eyes while talking on the phone) to get the truth or answers. Some do exercises to slow the breath down – this will allow you to connect to the intimate details of the truth.

Nadine, automatic writing with Gabrielle's comments—

How do we do this? No one taught me to do this. It's in my connect to do this.

Some can learn to slow their breath down through yoga, meditation classes, books, etc.

Lots of people could be connected to Abraham or our Gabrielle Collective. There is not a Biblical meaning behind any of the names. Names are only names.

It is so important that people be aware of what they can do. The growth of manifesting is important – it's not for our generation but future generations. How powerful it would be if everyone thought in the light. Pure mind over matter to change weather systems, to change technology. Literally an Act of God... *we have the ability to change these things, so that bad weather is out over the oceans all the time.*

I have faith I can give people faith in the unknown. *There are no words to describe how all powerful we are.* Hhhhmmm... have heart, have health, mercy Mercey me.

Why don't I have a cajillion dollars in the bank? Because I haven't worked to do that. *Faith, love, understanding, finding the balance are the rules of the game.*

Psychic realm... like sifting through the shoe sales rack of the store... some of it is garbage... it becomes confusing... *there is no one particular way – there are a lot of ways to read.*

Wanting to touch base with Aunt Helen [request for a client]. *Some can: the fact is it might be energies that the person requesting, what they are pulling out. The answer is something that you manifested... Aunt Helen doesn't stay as in her Sunday's best... she may opt to be a different energy... it doesn't make sense that she come back down here as how she was exactly when she left.*

The extreme energy is the message that comes through to give faith to help. A ricochet of energy from Aunt Helen. What that client needed at that time comes through... it might not be in Aunt Helen's typical wording. Most possible to get immediately after death the communication which needs to be dealt with.

What is innate wisdom? *It is when people are born with wisdom already intact, and abilities with attributes in their soul on this plane. We find ourselves in different physical worlds, hard relationships, lessons, for the purpose of connecting to your source. "To-be-downloaded" information is being supplied to each person to help with that person's plan or contract.* To be initially a good person is my vibration ... *downloaded info will be on real estate or banking – it is the information part of the parcel to take to your next job. You're still part of a collective source which is part of a universal source where our insight comes from!*

We awaken to all of this!

* * *

From Gabrielle—

There is a tendency to refer to the process of information transfer as 'channeling'. This is not correct in the case of communicating with us, via Donna. We are not channeling information through to her. This must be understood. Channeling is a term referring to when people make a connection with a particular energy, and since people are able to basically manifest anything they would like, channeling is not extremely dependable. Picking up energies is totally different, and understanding the vibrations of those energies is what is more feasible and possible. That is still not channeling. We do not channel information to Donna.

Our information is received by a 'connection'. Donna is connected to us. This is where she has obtained her wisdom from. She will always feel and speak the ways of Gabrielle collectively. Such is the way with others who have information. In common terms, Donna is an 'inside trader'.

You are part of us and you are connected to Donna. Yes, Nadine, you have been with us as well. All return to the Earthly plane with various attributes. One cannot take everything with them, for that would result in no growth at all. It is necessary to grow.

Donna has been given a personality in which many trust. She has also been given the wisdom and intelligence to make many listen. She is able to set an example and be followed. You have been given the gift of heal-

ing and amplifying awareness. You also have the ability to induce faith in those who have had little faith. You are both working on behalf of the collective, as are many others.

The connection with us vibrates continuously. It is simply functioning on a little higher level than most people, yet it seems as the path of least resistance to you and Donna alike. It is the path of least resistance, because it is who you are. Yes, we are able to guide you, via your own awareness, by way of affirmations, which in return, increase your faith, thus increasing your abilities to affect change.

It really doesn't matter as to what level those around you know of your connection with us. The fact is that there is a connection, as there is with Donna. Wisdom, truth, faith, love, compassion. It is from this arm of the Universal One that true peace can be obtained. Peace within yourself, and peace amongst each other.

All things are possible. Consider yourself blessed to remember your connection to us, and to receive our guidance. Not all have done this. You left the collective with the knowledge that you could move mountains. Remember? You left with the knowledge that all things are possible. We cannot foresee the future, however we can certainly guide you in a path that you can make your future exactly what you'd like it to be. The future is yours.

So, in closing, once again, we do not channel *information. You are part of us, as we are part of you. Donna is simply the connection, and the teachings and words coming from us through her is merely her ability to vibrate at a frequency which allows the passage of this wisdom and assistance. Information does not get channeled to you. You already know this information, you are simply getting the information affirmed by Donna, thereby remembering it, which in turn makes it true to you. Donna's energy is here to help people make light of life. To help them along their journey with faith and courage. She is strong in her connection, as you are.*

Take care,

Gabrielle et al

Who are all these angels? Bellum is female and is my guardian angel.

My son Eric just reconfirmed this and didn't recall saying that 9 years ago. She is light blue and pink, Eric says, and she comes and goes, but he doesn't know where she goes. She goes and talks to other angels for me (she's not a listed archangel); she is a specific angel to me (not a connecting angel), he explained. She helps me and prepares me and gives me defenses when I need them. Bellum is a protector to me and my children.

I asked Eric does she have any special abilities, like healing? He says, "D'uh! She's *your* angel...."

When I asked about Shurean (mentioned at the end of a message from Gabrielle), Eric said that's a foreign drug that hippies use. *lol* He doesn't know.

Jonathon? I believe Donna talks to him to get messages; she talks to my angels. Eric doesn't know who Jonathon is. When I go inside and ask, they say he talks to me all the time. They just said he is a connecting angel to help others. Everyone has a connecting angel – that's how I get the information about a specific person. It seems I talk to their angel or angels and I translate what they are saying.

Apparently, according to several psychics, I use the archangels all the time. Honestly, I dunno. I never called on them specifically by name to ask for anything.

Okay, the boys are rowdy here. Getting ready for bed. Can't concentrate... Hope that helps you understand.

Tommy James sings 'Draggin' The Line'
I feel fine
I'm talkin' 'bout peace of mind
I'm gonna take my time
I'm gettin' the good sign
Draggin' the line

This was Tommy's comeback solo hit after nearly dying of drug abuse. The term 'dragging the line' is similar to the saying 'towing the line'. Tommy is fine, his state of mind was good and he would be patient for whatever came his way.

CHAPTER 24

Becoming healed

I want to tell a story about curing myself – with Sharon's encouragement, and energy – and what I learned (or, as Gabrielle would say, what I remembered).

During my yearly check up, my medical doctor asks me if I was still selling real estate. This seemed a loaded question because I believe she knew I wasn't selling real estate full-time anymore – we've had conversations before about my abilities.

We got into discussing the healing career that I was embarking on, and she was asking questions like "how do you know the energy gets to that person and doesn't hit someone else instead?" Maybe she was imagining a gun shooting silver energy bullets to blast away disease.

She was trying to quantify things based on her education as to how this could be real. "How can a girl from Brantford in a short period of time have such a big shift – that's amazing!" she said.

She wasn't asking questions as a person who wanted to know for the benefit of helping people, or that we could help each other to help people. She never asked what type of people do you see, what can you do, how many have you treated. I've never received a referral from her. It was apparent she wanted not to talk about it further at this time, as it upset her world view. I respected her level of awareness just the same.

Then out of the blue she decides that she wants to re-examine an x-ray of two years ago that showed I had fibroids. "Oh, your fibroids were getting big. We should have an ultrasound."

I am grateful and was looking forward to an ultrasound – was this an affirmation that I had forgotten myself? Did I need to pay more attention to what was going on in my own life? I certainly wasn't aware of any symptoms.

You see, two years ago she referred me to a specialist to possibly have the fibroids removed surgically. I was in much pain and discomfort, and got frustrated with the system waiting six months for an appointment. So I meditated to try to heal myself, the symptoms went away and the case was dropped then by the specialist when I told him I didn't have any issues to deal with. The specialist let me go. He was of East Indian descent and understood, it seemed, that healing happens in many ways.

A few days after this latest visit with my family practitioner, I met Sharon and she sensed a spot (exactly where the fibroid was located). She said I should continue working on it – she could work towards helping me. She felt she could move this along for me. She also felt I could finish what I started, I just needed to be aware that my work wasn't finished. I had forgot about myself while I was healing others.

As a result Sharon and I did get together for one healing session in addition to my healing myself by creative visualization, using castor oil packs and soaking in high vibrational detox baths. I could feel energy coming out of my abdomen. I noticed I was calmer and more peaceful than before; I did recall that certain feelings towards a previous relationship just disappeared.

My ultrasound was then taken. There was no follow up call from the doctor. As healers we tend to believe there is a spiritual remedy for everything. I needed to do a little mental housekeeping and look into my past to filter out those learned behaviors. I needed to give more affirmation of self-love and respect, and to overcome my negative beliefs.

I brought this ailment on through my thoughts, and my body was talking to me to let something go. I needed to release the pain in my thoughts and let go of the patterns that caused the body to give me a sign to pay attention to what was in my heart and what was in my head.

Louise Hay, in her book *You Can Heal Your Life*, states that fibroids come from nursing hurt from a partner, a blow to the feminine ego. (I had one bad relationship after another it seemed.) Louise teaches to give yourself affirmation to release the pattern in you that created this experience. Affirm that you *only create good in your life*.

I learned to ask for protection to release this matter that caused stress and inflammation in my body. The energy had released in the area that I was holding on to it. So did my obsessions about others' thoughts that I allowed to come into me.

Emailed advice from Donna—

You're suffering from *energy depletion*, and I've got this message for you before… or maybe part of the message.

We'll call your own energy simply *energy*. And we'll call the energy that you receive for healing *cosmic medicine*. If you were responsible for giving me cosmic medicine pills every day, and always had some pills left over, would you eat them? Or take them back to the pharmacy? I think you have caught the drift.

Now your energy: it is necessary that you rid yourself of doubt, especially with the relationship with Mike. That wears on your energy. If it's not fun, and not good – don't do it! Smile, laugh and be merry. Separate healing from living. Send your residual patient concerns to the higher power and Universe to be looked after.

Make sure that when people leave your house, that you ask that *their* energy be detached from yours. Their soul may not like it, but it will be done. This will prevent getting dragged down and any form of vibrational pressures you get. I think that this may be happening. When you see a person for a healing, they need you and as you make them feel better, their energy automatically feels good and then attaches onto yours. You allow this to happen unconsciously, because you are healing them. Then, when they leave, they are still attached, even though the physical distance may be great. Your energy is sensitive, and maybe even allergic to this interaction, since it's at a much different vibration – kind of like A positive blood and B negative blood. That will produce a reaction, similar to an allergy. You may heat up, you may get cold, you make shake or vibrate. You may feel sick. Just asking for this separation isn't quite enough – right now. You must visualize a stream of energy coming out of them and attaching onto you, just like an octopus's tentacle, and then you must visualize yourself, taking your hand, pulling it off and giving it back. This will help you tremendously. Think of when someone takes a child to school for the first day, and they cling on to your skirt. Would you leave the school with their hand still attached to your skirt? No, because you know that the hand would be attached to their little body! So, you would remove their hand – that's what it's like.

Remember: every single thing occurs to aid us in our Universal Growth. If we don't understand it, or don't absorb it, it simply keeps recurring until we do understand it or absorb it. When we get it, then we can move on. It's all in moving us to a higher level! Smile, laugh and grow!

Donna, with more advice—

Mike is a *real* person. Perhaps he vibrates on a level that I can communicate with, whatever it is, he's good! Cast aside *your insecurities now!* You're beautiful, you're fun… and there's no other person that he'd rather spend time with! Furthermore… *lol* … he's into you for all the right reasons. He's not around you to suck every ounce of energy, he's got huge energy himself, he's into you for growth and love. It's very good.

Testimonial just in—

Nadine, I visited you at your house a little while back. CS— had recommended me to you. I thought you should know that almost everything you said was true and if it hadn't happened then it has by now. You really have a gift.

Thanks so much.

– M— in Florida

&

Mike calls and says, "What did you do to me? All the things I did before that I thought made me happy, I don't want to do them any more. I'm not the same person. Everyone is noticing."

The doctor warned him that he was headed for a stroke. But now his blood pressure is down for the first time in five years. His doctor is amazed.

Mike volunteers the dirt: "I don't want to drag the line and chase skirts. I haven't in weeks. What did you do to me?"

I answered, "Nothing that you didn't ask for. You called for me, I came into your life as you wanted help."

"Those days are gone," Mike says. He looks at things differently, he has more patience with people and doesn't get upset as easily. He's more of a negotiator instead of a fighter. A feared martial arts expert, he now walks away from conflict instead of seeking it.

The addictions, the things that caused large gaps between us, have subsided. Mike said that he has one ounce left of Vodka in a bottle at home and that would be the last ounce he would use to pledge to let go towards a new beginning.

Mike was sexually abused by a male at the tender age of 12. He had a early childhood relationship at home that haunted him for years. Mike left home at the age of 15 to go live with his grandmother. At 17 he was out on his own. Running away from himself, traveling the world connecting to others, building relationships to help others and protect others it seems but never sustained a relationship long enough to settle down in marriage. Mike feared not knowing how to love himself.

Mike is 52 years of age and asks this question often: *How come I never married?* Twelve months ago he pushed the blame on others. Now he sees and is more aware of what he always has been. Now he is ready to shine.

In a card Mike wrote me six months ago, he said, "Thank you for opening my heart so I can feel / for opening my eyes so I can see / for opening my soul so I can live / love always – Mike."

This was my affirmation Mike was feeling guilt in his life about the things he had done, the hurt he inflicted on others. By running, he was rejecting himself – he felt inadequate to be a partner with someone else. Many times I had to be kind and clear and teach him how to respect. The 3,000 miles between us made our hearts grow stronger. (A little intuition helped too – I could see him from a distance and could believe Mike was making progress.)

The space allowed us each to grow in our own lives doing what we needed to accomplish. We were growing independently of each other without being co-dependant living together day by day. The distance was definitely good.

Mike's friends and family could see big changes in Mike and realized I was the positive influence that Mike needed in his life at this time. So many woman before tried to change him, he said, but he never chose to listen. Mike said, how can you possibly be accepted into my circle of friends I've had for 30 years so quickly? Why you?

Mike started asking the *why* question. I knew when he did he was asking and believing for change in himself. I gave him space and affirmation to believe in himself. He would call me in the middle of the night to interpret his vivid dreams. That was an affirmation he was reaching out for help, and my belief was that his dreams reflected progress – his letting go of his fears and learned behaviors. We would have new beginnings together.

He is now discovering how wonderful he is, he has chosen to love and enjoy himself. He is living in the *Now*. Each moment is new for Mike. He likes and approves of his changes. Now he was becoming ready to love another how he would want to be loved in return.

When we first met, the first thing Mike said was he was the first person ever who would accept me for who I am. That stuck and played in my head. Was I not awake then, was I living to be someone else for other people's approval? Mike taught me to ground myself, as he watched over for me from a distance. He taught me to be me. Mike gave me clarity when I couldn't see. He gave me belief to keep going on my path.

This storytelling guy has a charmed life! The people from all walks of life – philosophers, doctors, bartenders, call girls, Mohammad Ali, Chuck Norris, Sylvester Stallone, real hired hitman, the Russian Mafia, Hell's Angels – he had a full life and everyone loved Mike it seemed. Why do I have to meet these colorful people? Somehow it is part of my life's plan. These stories are meant to be told so others could stop and relate to the consequences of our thoughts and reactions.

We all need to share our gifts to learn from each other. When I tried to walk away from the lessons, he said, "That's fine, but I am just suppose to always love you and watch out over you to protect you."

Mike has gone through a major awakening and shift. Kinda magical, really. I knew he had it in him but didn't think his shift would be coming so soon. Not to be overanxious (because I still have to see more to believe it can last) but his friends and family are seeing a big difference and wanting this for the two of us. Gosh, his mother just bought Mike and I a trip to Hawaii to celebrate his healings and new beginnings!

My dreams that I had weeks ago confirm what I see in the day. Dunno, could be a longer relationship than I anticipated…

All in all, it's still the truth (which is the single most important thing anyone can do *every day* – tell the truth for others to learn from). Can people change? I say yes, if they want to. How do you get them to change? You can be kind and clear and let them make choices. Mike chose to come across to the light side.

There's still *lots* of room for growth for both of us, I'm sure. So we are still learning from each other so that we may help others. And there are definitely more doors and opportunities to open for each of us – this relationship seems to balance out, as difficult as it seems at times.

I'll fly out to see Mike this weekend. We are going for dinner with Henry and Nick in Vancouver Friday night. Maybe go to Victoria or stay in a cabin north of Whistler….

Mike said in his next life he wanted to come back as a real-life angel to help people. I said he *is* an angel because he helped and angeled me. "Oh, I hear the bell ringing as someone just got his wings." *lol*

The world around us just seems to be conspiring to keep us together (it's been a year).

Damn, it's hard to *read* for myself at times. And it's so easy to read for others.

※

At their seminar, I got a firm affirmation from Abraham and Esther about me being on the right track with my teachings. She repeated conversations about energy healers and repeated over and over five times: "Think It. Feel It. Share It."

That's exactly what I'd had printed on my business card. Since that seminar I have been in a very high vortex of energy – the flow is here and kicking up again. I'm very clear and focused!

※

Pat, my client in the hospital, was off the chart in energy level today. The nurses stopped me and started to cry and hug me to ask how I felt he was doing.

He has been in the hospital for over a year following a heart attack and stroke. He is now kicking his blankets off his bed (before he couldn't move his legs).

He turned his head and looked at me, then smiled and reached out for my hand – not once but four times upon request he repeated this. He reached out to his wife Lisa from a distance. We laughed and laughed, out loud with tears in our eyes!!!

Pat *is* getting stronger and growing inside every day. His soul *never* waivered while his body was paralyzed. In fact, his vibration is rising daily as he learns through the challenges. What an example he sets for us all about becoming aware, to grow in love and balance.

※

Contemplating my past relationships with men again. I now know that we're all on this Earth to learn from each other. There are different lessons we each must learn, in each relationship. Previous lovers seem to have learned a wee bit, but mostly hadn't gotten the lessons. Prince Harming likely will not get his lessons in this lifetime – he's far too caught up in control and financial wealth (which he can't separate). With him I learned to be my own self, and to protect myself from another person's darkness.

The pattern of relationships continued right up to Mike. I learned to speak clearly and be kind, and he chose to heal himself in many ways. He actually received the most benefit of all the men I have dated. My internal affirmation is clear on that. Whether or not we continue to date one more month from now or not, he did chose to make a large improvement in his life for the better. He can see now and is still learning.

Angels and friends alike want me to bring Mike into this more – saying he has turned the corner and gives hope for others. He can show men and women alike that people can change – it's never too late. We are all divine.

Mike is very open in telling the world what a schmuck he's been and how he is wanting so hard to be a better person. Again, if you tell your truth, ask and believe in yourself, you will have success. You can't change what you are not aware of. Telling your truth builds awareness and clarity. Telling one's truth is the most important thing you can do. It will set you free.

I want us all to reflect on our past, present and future relationships. Romance ties in clearly with your self-love aspect. If you love yourself, you can get through anything. The recipe requires a dash of love, an ounce of respect, a pinch of togetherness – to be loved just like everyone wants.

Did I forget to mention adding in some laughter? Out loud and often? *lol*

MUSIC TRACK
Van Halen performing 'Dreams'
We belong in a world that must be strong
Oh, that's what dreams are made of

CHAPTER 25

Dreams of destiny

September 17 08, journal entry—
Last week I had another night of headaches, restlessness. So intense and painful many would go to the hospital or take pharmaceuticals, but I concentrated on being calm and waiting it out.

Now realizing that this power is far bigger than I'd thought – tied to all aspects of the Earth and its people and physical tension. Was getting some message of significant events brewing.

Next morning turned on TV to see what happened. Nothing in particular. The following morning was the stock market meltdown. My savings are so little that this isn't a big deal for us.

So I'd had ample warning and signs to move my own savings out of stocks, but hadn't interpreted it. Can feel another – bigger – stock market event coming very soon.

The market went back up 800 points – whew, saved by the bell! I went immediately to the bank that day and was *told* to put it all in money markets. The market did crash again several times. I was saved.

❧

27 September 08, journal entry—
I dream a lot. The kind where you see in color, you feel the emotions,

you see the symbolisms clearly, you can go into the dream, interpret as you go and can change the dream as some would call lucid dreaming. I've heard about people dreaming where they are flying – for the first time I can say I've experienced this phenomenon. This dream had a message for me to interpret to others.

It was night time and on Earth people were dying, the blood in the dream was very clear. Innocent people were being hurt and they didn't understand why. The ones to escape the energies that hurt others considered themselves to be fortunate or lucky to be alive.

These energies causing the tragedies could not see me but they knew I existed. I knew the source of this energy was trying to find me too. I waited patiently and didn't know what would happen, although I knew I needed to make a difference and help many on Earth. I needed to understand how to escape them first before trying to explain to people the questions that they had of me.

I looked up to the night sky and could see little balls of white light traveling in packs and floating down to Earth. We all knew they existed, they couldn't hide their appearances to me, others knew they existed but couldn't see them. The human race is conscious of their harm. All of us also wanted to escape from their harm.

I remember the feeling of jumping up into the sky high above and away from the source of energy. I was given the knowledge that all we had to do was to ask to be invisible. We could actually hide from these energies that targeted at us. All we had to do was ask. However the energies could never hide from us.

My physical body would fly back down to Earth to raise those who didn't know how to ask for help. I would speak to their souls and rescue them. They were grateful. I remember the feeling of power of being stronger than the inflicting energies that were trying to harm the Earth. I woke up and realized I had remembered the feelings of flying and of doing good on Earth. We could teach others to fly, to become invisible and protected from the harmful energies.

What I didn't understand while waking was *what were these energies?* Can we define them? Should we? I remembered the harm these energies inflicted upon Earth. Were they *dark energies?* Is there such a thing as dark energy? There is so much still for me to learn.

Halfway through the next day, the dream played out over and over in my head. I turned to Gabrielle for clarity – I phoned Donna to connect me with the Gabrielle Collective.

Donna didn't know about my dream of the light balls in the sky. I asked her simply *is there such thing as dark energy?* Here is her reply from Gabrielle:

All energy is pure. All energy is good as it shines down from Source, it is absolutely pure white energy when it's received. The energy you speak of, that being so-called Dark, is remnant or residual Earth energy. Just like a snowball, it takes on the shape and form of those who pass it on. Negative dark Earthbound energy can be washed clean by Source energy, and if captured can be directed back to Source for cleansing and forgiveness.

A few hours later I went into a dress shop to speak to my friend Kathryn. She is also a connection and had a message for me: *There is no such thing as dark energy. Others will ridicule you about your knowledge as it conflicts with the knowledge they have been taught. Keep going and don't give up hope. You will help many to understand.*

She had tears in her eyes and a warm hug for my knowledge. (Kathryn didn't know what I dreamt last night and that I was looking for clarity, yet her soul knew.)

With the support of all my dear friends and family, I will keep following the signs, those angel tracks into the light.

With love,
– Nadine Mercey

MUSIC TRACK
Children's entertainment superstar Fred Penner tells us to be 'Proud'
[more at www.fredpenner.com]
You've got to be proud
Of the people around you
Proud of the things that you do
Proud of your dreams and feelings inside you
Never afraid to let them shine through

BONUS CHAPTER 1

Manifesting

The word *manifesting* has leapt into popular culture with books such as *The Secret* and *The Power of Intention,* and the speeches of Dr. Wayne Dyer and others. Yes, you really can influence future events – by praying or concentrating and asking for a specific result – but what exactly happens may surprise you. My friend was CEO of a large multinational and quite unhappy about never spending time with his family both physically and mentally – the business seemed to suck away all his energy and attention so he seemed spaced out and preoccupied even when with his wife and son. He began to earnestly hope for a career change. Sure enough that soon came, but in the form of being dismissed by the directors, followed by a 16-month-long, bitter court battle over severance pay. Eventually, he won the legal battle, but not before learning life lessons in humility, patience and forgiveness. These were teachings watched over by his angels, all were pre-ordained challenges in his life's contract. What he'd manifested was a way that he – and his opponents in the lawsuits – would be presented with learning opportunities.

You see, you can't really change your overall life plan; you must learn the lessons that you came to this planet to learn.

As long as the asked-for thing or change is for the *highest and best interest*, it can come about. But if you are asking for material things in particular, or ego-based power trips, you may get what you sought, wrapped up in a very rough lesson. Be careful.

Following are tips for increasing the effectiveness of your manifesting.

1. *Believe* that your thoughts shape your reality. If you don't think manifesting positive outcomes works, it probably won't for you. But be aware that deeply believing in negative events can be a form of manifesting those outcomes. Remember that *worry is a prayer for disaster.* I teach my healing clients to open up and believe. The energy does sink in more; the quantity and process is quicker, and the results are longer-lasting.

2. Get *connected* – realize that you are not separate from your desire, so imagine and *experience* yourself receiving your intention now.

3. Become *clear* about your desires – visualize the details.

4. Be *open to receiving* – feel you are truly worthy and deserving of receiving your intention.

5. Let go of the *how*. Once you've set an intention, it's time for trust and faith to set in. When you put a cake in the oven, you don't question that it will bake. And it ruins the cake if you doubt and open the oven door every two minutes to check.

6. Be *unattached* to the outcome. Life will unfold in its perfect order. When we are too attached to a specific outcome and timeline, the energy becomes restricted and we cut off the natural flow. Take this advice from The Beatles: *Let it be.*

For clients or participants in a workshop who need to raise their awareness or to believe in the ability to send energy, I will do a quick exercise to help them open up to the opportunity. I send energy from a distance and they feel it instantly – then they believe. You only get what you believe. The first healing is great but the second is even greater!

You each have the power of inner choice! We are all searching for the *hidden* truth! Why not think about developing your intuition as I have? You get to be creative. You could hear the messages, feel the energy, see the dreams become reality. You get to decide!

MUSIC TRACK
George Michaels performing 'Faith'
I reconsider
My foolish notion
I need someone to hold me
But I'll wait for something more
You've got to believe.

BONUS CHAPTER 2

Control: Ego and spirit

The ego has a vibration just as the spirit does.

Control comes out of ego which is driven by fear.

Spirit comes from within and can be brought in.

On one end of the scale is fear. Fear has a frequency brought in by our thoughts. At the other end is the love frequency which also comes from thoughts.

In the book *Power vs. Force: The Hidden Determinants of Human Behavior* [ISBN 978-1561709335], Dr. David R. Hawkins says in his intro, "Man thinks he lives by virtue of the forces he can control, but in fact he's governed by power from unrevealed sources."

His research suggests we can be on one side of the scale to have thought forms and experience a frequency of shame, guilt, apathy, grief, fear, on up to desire, anger, pride and courage. But you can also further increase your vibration to trust, willingness, acceptance, reason, love – and on to joy then peace, to the ultimate vibration of enlightenment where you experience the ultimate divine energy, receiving it and giving it! The further you rise up the vibration scale the stronger the body will be to combat disease and receiving information for truth.

197

You will get through life's little surprises a whole lot easier if you surrender to the positive vibes and let go of the control and fear.

Don't surrender the dreams. Instead surrender the one thing you
don't have and never will: *control*.

These may all seem so complex or theoretical to some who want improvement. If you can remember one thing when times seem hard: go
to your *I-am* presence – find an environment that makes you feel good.
Do a hobby, take up golf or knitting, and meditate if you can't get into
yoga. Do something that pleasures you to stay in that positive vibration.
Remember positive vibes attract positive movements in your evolving
life, even without you knowing.

Just how do we know when to surrender? It's simple: our physical
body gives us signals to warn us that earlier energy entered (maybe
unconsciously with someone else's or our intent or not) and there was
a competition for energy. We need to pay attention to the warning signals – they are there, bad feelings or good feelings. If there is a physical
ailment, chances are the energy entered into the subconscious, unconscious, super conscious, delta, alpha, beta, theta, and all the other seven
brains of the body.

We can be aware of the physical problems that cause us to reach out
for help. However we aren't always aware of mind thoughts or string
energies stored in the body most of your life which may manifest into
sickness much later. For example, I had a 46-year-old client who had
thought-form energies stored in his physical body since he was in the
mother's womb. As a psychic, this information was channeled to me. I
visually created a way to speak to his soul (his true self) to unlock that
energy. Again visualizing my colorful dots and belief system, I pushed
and pulled the energy pattern as I was guided to, building awareness
and sending energy to those areas that were affected. After the healing
he felt relieved and renewed – almost *reborn*. The physical ailments instantly dissipated. Old thought patterns were recognized and discard-
ed with kindness by the client, making room for clarity and purpose in
his new beliefs.

As he recognized healthier choices and increased his vibration levels,
others around him soon felt the love as well. Life got much easier for
this individual, and he could help others.

MUSIC TRACK
Listen to T'pau singing 'Heart and Soul'
Something in the moonlight catches my eye
... Give a little bit of heart and soul
... Give a sign I need to know

BONUS CHAPTER 3

Nadinisms

These are statements I say day to day. While I do love quoting others, a few of these Nadinisms just popped into my mind, from past lives and angels unknown.

- Believe you can feel good about yourself even when at that moment you don't. Like a spatula and a bowl, scoop away all those adverse thoughts, and allow the energy of your collective universe to get into your skin. Let go to the magic of the rhythm, to the reason, the dance and your space.
- The fear brings on hard lessons to teach them to surrender to get over their fears. Know what you want and live it. Transpire your wishes into health.
- "Everything is worship if your mind is focused on the present moment." – Paulo Coelho
- The teacher never tells the student what he or she *should* do.
- Know love. "Love fills everything. It cannot be desired because it is an end in itself. It cannot betray because it has nothing to do with possession. It cannot be held prisoner because it is a river and will overflow its banks. Anyone who tries to imprison love will cut off the spring that feeds it." — Paulo Coelho

- Simply put, there is fear and love. Any emotion in between is a cover for fear or love. You get to decide: will I live in a hostile environment in myself or a positive one?
- Inner peace: my moments of indecision, my desire to simply live in peace, to be the slave of my feelings and to surrender myself without asking any questions, without even knowing if my love is reciprocated. Awaken the goddess in all of us... everything is a part of the goddess. Everything is one.
- To change: re-program yourself every minute of each day, to thoughts that make you grow. Ask, receive and believe your intentions are real.
- We may be witnessing a very important moment in history of the world, when the spirit finally merges with the material, and the two are united and transformed.
- Now: I'm learning to teach people. Ironically, you've got to teach them what you don't know, and listen to make them know what they themselves are gifted to teach. This is teaching people to grow.
- You can't see past the choices you haven't made.
- You've got to breathe – to go within and allow the energy to flow through you till you involuntary vibrate and allow the power to come within.
- We're not alone on the paths we follow, we bump into paths of others.
- Laugh at your worries and insecurities because life is full of mystery. It's important to have a sense of humor. *lol*
- Believe.
- "You give little when you give your possessions. It is when you give yourself that you truly give." – Paulo Coelho
- It's about connecting the dots, filling in the spaces, finding the inner love and finding the forgiveness of past and present life.
- In your blood is what you are now. The instinct I have knows the dance, the song, the laughter, the ability to bring the vortex high to receive the energy to flow through the hands to heal.
- Only fear of fate separates us and pulls us apart. Cry, release the fear and move ahead!
- Your thoughts are things.

- All in all, realize the importance of allowing fate and of welcoming opportunities for people to come into your life.
- There are no coincidences. You've just got to connect the dots with love, patience and kindness.
- More power = more wisdom = more love for all to give and receive. We are powerful conduits of what has been lost but *now* found.... The physical tells us so.
- Why are we sick? To remind us we are well at heart – just wake up and see.
- We can't control beyond what we need, so we get what we receive as we know it. We will never be able to control beyond our destiny. To learn, to live, to love, to share are the actions of truth.
- Knowledge isn't the same as wisdom; wisdom is *doing* it.
- Are you happy? Happy has to do with everything!
- Why can't you sleep at night? Grab a pen and paper and write it down. *They* are trying to talk to you.
- Awareness... A state of mind. That's all it is.
- My job is service to others, to help teach.
- People are hungry for the truth, a better and easier way to see clearly.
- Slow down – you might taste something.
- Learn from your own life experience without eating sloppily.
- Start gathering information outside yourself, although the only place you'll find what you need is on the inside.
- Fear: suddenly everything seems so empty.
- You want to be more, to be someone who uses his mind and body in ways most people never dreamed of. I can teach you.
- People aren't their thoughts. They think they are, and that brings them sadness.
- The mind is a reflex organ, it reacts to everything.
- Developing the right wisdom: to develop the wisdom in the right place, in the right time.
- Emptying our minds takes a lifetime of practice, and takes you out of your mind too.
- The mind fills up again and misses everything that's going on.

- When you are truly in the here and now, it's amazing what you can do!
- Find your process to clear your mind. How long did you stay that way? Ego comes back, to gloat on your progress, not in the Now, saying that you haven't learned anything.
- For the healers and those being healed: I have had to learn to respect that this is all they know and to respect their level of awareness.
- We can listen to others' thoughts – have you ever stopped to listen?
- Sometimes you have to lose your mind before you come to your senses.
- Step outside yourself and view you.
- Healers: send people away till they are ready to learn more. People need to trust their healer/teacher. They have to be strong in order to be awake.
- Meditate in every action.
- Clean up your addictions to knowing everything when you know nothing.
- All you have is right *now!*
- Pay attention to the hard moments. As hard as they are, they bring joy, peace, love and enlightenment.
- Hanging on for dear life, afraid to fall? Not giving up anything, nothing you lost, what are you holding on to? See yourself, the one you have to let go of.
- If you don't know who you are without knowing, then what are you doing?
- Emotions are natural – it's life passing wind.
- Everything has a purpose, even this. Up to you to find it.
- Anger, hatred, violence – it is just fear.
- People hardest to love are usually the ones who need it the most.
- Stop and think. Then you see love, recognize true love. And you will inspire and aspire for it.
- There is never *nothing* going on. There are no ordinary moments, now you have learned.
- Celebrate!
- There is no better. You will never be better. Same as you will never

be less than anyone else. The habit is the problem. All you have to do is to be conscious of your choice and responsible for your actions.

- You chose me. How do you know I am not your intuition speaking to you right now?
- Every action has its price and pleasure. Be responsible for yours.
- Give freely to the Takers. They will get what they are taking.
- Apologize.
- Don't be sloppy with your life. When you feel fear, use the sword, cut the mind ribbons, slash the regrets and fears.
- Devote your life to your higher purpose.
- He who finds the love in what he does, doesn't give up.
- It is not about perfection, it's about absolute vulnerability.
- Train to do what you are meant to do.
- When others give up on you, don't give up on yourself.
- If you don't get what you want, you suffer. When you get exactly what you want, you still suffer, because you can't hold on to it forever.
- Don't surrender the dreams. Surrender the one thing you don't have and never will… control.
- You may or you may not. You are something exceptional either way.
- Living in fear that you might fear?
- You can't deposit pride and prejudice in the bank.
- Then when you're finally ready to see – it's a long hike.
- Life's 3 rules—
  1. *Paradox*. Life is a mystery, don't waste time figuring it out.
  2. *Humor*. Keep a sense of humor especially about yourself.
  3. *Change*. Nothing stays the same.
- The journey is what brings us happiness, not the destination.
- How far we have come! Don't let anyone stop you from your journey, from what you want and need to do.
- Show them. Show yourself.
- Dream stuff. Sometimes it comes true. Maybe it will.
- Whatever you learn, others will want that magic rubbed off on them.
- You make every move about the move, not about what others think.
- Getting everything you want is not about the vision of winning.

- Star is a maker. A maker is a star. You are a star maker, so dream on.
- Find your presence. Fill yourself up with warm and loving compassion. For me the best way to meditate and enter into contact with the light was by knitting. My Grandmother taught me through repetition and harmony. We learn to creatively visualize the power of intent. I was now lost in my own world without being a victim. Most of us are not meant for solitude, and we only know ourselves when we see ourselves in the eyes of others. By finding your *I-am* presence, you increase your velocity and in return your dimension as the Earth prepares for its increase to a higher dimension.
- Awaken the repressed energy inside when you feel that push-pull feeling. For example, walk down the street and say, "I'm here and now."
- Sit for a few minutes each day and do nothing... getting as much out of that time as you can, just *being*.
- It's a simple matter of being aware: that we can be silent and can open to a greater energy – through creative visualization.
- Learn from everyone you can who walks into your life, and surrender to the lessons of self-worth and knowledge. This wisdom is the most powerful form of enlightenment one can do for yourself – and, yes, higher than meditation.
- Just keep flowing the paths of life, live in the moment and always remember: "There is no way to happiness, happiness *is* the way."
- Find love in small deeds.
- Protect yourself and do build barriers.
- Engage the Spiritual darkness.
- Ask for the highest and best purpose. Creatively visualize the energy leaving and/or entering your body.
- Believe. More. Trust.
- Read positive influential books. Go for a walk. Listen to music and bring out the dance of your vortex.
- Be clear and kind when teaching the lesson.
- Know when you say *I love you* that love can be of many forms.
- Share your stories and gifts with others often.
- Prune regularly.
- Finished learning the lesson? Then the teacher is gone. *lol*

Kim Mitchell singing 'Bad Times'
Artists write songs for their own healings –
and also to teach others through their lyrics.

Learning from 'Bad Times'

Out of intense personal relationship challenges, sometimes great creativity emerges. We learn and we grow in awareness. My friend Kim Mitchell never reveals the inspiration for his song lyrics, preferring to let the listener use their imagination, yet I wonder if he wrote these powerful lyrics as a message... something about us?

BAD TIMES

She's a total disaster in the first degree
A pair of high-heeled blues waiting just for me
The lights are red and the money's blue
She lives down by the railroad avenue
The same old dance steps to the same old song
Take a one way ride... it doesn't last too long
It's a lifetime sentence and no one ever gets free
Because she got the diamonds... and I got disease

Might as well laugh 'cause you can't dance
When you're on your knees... begging for mercy

I can see you're havin' bad times
Ooooo so bad... nothing rhymes
I can see you're havin' bad times
Only one more line before it starts to unwind
I can see you're havin' bad times
So bad so bad so bad... nothing rhymes

I can see you're havin' bad times
She's like a lying politician at election time

Front page headline and it's all bad news
A stiletto-heeled version of the walking blues
All fancy wrapping but nothing's inside
There's no bargain prices for a downhill ride
Sweet sweet poison dressed in ermine and lace
And the weatherman's calling for champagne and rain
Always center stage at the scene of the crime
A cruel joke dressed up just like a valentine

So you might as well laugh 'cause you can't dance
When you're on your knees... begging for mercy

I can see you're havin' bad times
Ooooo so bad... nothing rhymes
I can see you're havin' bad times
She's no misdemeanor... she's a felony crime
I can see you're havin' bad times
Ooooo so bad so bad... nothing rhymes
I can see you're havin' bad times
One day in her bad books is like doing hard time

Funny how you always want it... just one more time
When she wins... that's when you lose
On a good day you'll walk away
Still wearing your old shoes

I can see you're havin' bad times
Oh so bad... nothing rhymes
I can see you're havin' bad times
She's all fancy wrapping but nothing's inside
I can see you're havin' bad times
There ain't no bargain prices for a downhill ride

I can see you're havin' bad times
Ooooo so bad
I can see you're havin' bad times
She's all fancy wrapping but nothing's inside
I can see you're havin' bad times
Ooooo so bad so bad... nothing rhymes
I can see you're havin' bad times.

Kim Mitchell did learn something from me – to laugh out loud as much as possible even when you can't dance.

Kim and I always had a real cool connection where we respected each other's lives, even when we couldn't understand at that moment. *lol* We'll always be friends to guide each other. What's uncanny is we both wrote about our souls mentioning each other's shoes. He is famous for those Converse shoes – you should have seen how many shoes this man has!!!! *You Rawk, Kim!*

ABOUT THE AUTHOR

NADINE MERCEY is a high vibrational healer.

She grew up in Brantford, Ontario, and confesses to having never done well at formal education. "My mind just didn't work like other people's." Looking back, she recognizes signs of mild autism in her behavior.

For twenty years, Nadine worked in real estate, rising to become one of Canada's top realtors. Her success came from an uncanny ability to intuitively understand the needs and motivations of buyers and sellers. Her awakening to the extent of her intuitive capabilities came from selling a haunted house – one that had been featured in her dreams since childhood.

Soon she was experiencing great vibrational development – and receiving messages in her mind from voices who identified themselves as angels. She is guided and protected by the Gabrielle Collective and other energies.

Nadine conducts readings, often at great distances, during which she communicates with the client's spirit guide(s) and/or angel(s). These entities provide instruction about what is required to raise the person's vibration, in order to restore balance to soul, mind and body.

Generally energy flows into the person's body as Nadine visualizes areas that need help. Healing happens through creative visualization, and only when intended *for the highest and best interest* – to help that person progress toward his or her predetermined life purpose.

Blessed with extraordinarily high vibration, Nadine devotes a portion of her practice to healing other intuitives and to making people aware of their own intuitive capabilities. She is a medical intuitive, who has helped doctors identify illnesses in their patients.

Nadine is a dynamic presenter at seminars, and has been the subject of a documentary film. Discussions are underway about hosting a television show. She is also developing her own line of healing products.

Nadine lives in Ancaster, Ontario, Canada with her two teenaged sons, Eric and Jaxon. She loves to dance and laugh. And she does own way too many shoes.

Her website is at *www.NadineMercey.com*

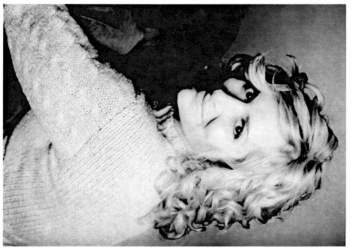

DONNA SANTOS
PHOTOGRAPHY

Please go to *www.NadineMercey.com* to follow the ever-evolving story of Nadine's life and career.

Her mission is to raise awareness about the potential in all of us to boost our personal vibration so we can be healthy, in loving relationships and following our pre-destined life path. *Have heart, have health* is her mantra.

Nadine is available as a presenter at conferences and fairs, and for interviews on radio and TV, and in print. She is developing seminars to help people awaken to higher vibrational awareness, and possibly become healers themselves.

To arrange a personal consultation, please contact Nadine through her website: *www.NadineMercey.com*

CPSIA information can be obtained at www.ICGtesting.com
Printed in the USA
LVOW11s2300240316

480609LV00001BA/108/P